to [signature]

May Yoga come to the rescue of our aching bones! — love,

Jill Coleman

WATERYOGA

Water-Assisted Postures and Stretches
for
Flexibility and Well-Being

by

Jill Coleman

Eglantine Press
Owings Mills, MD, U.S.A.
1998

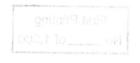

WATERYOGA

Publisher's Cataloging-in-Publication
(Provided by Quality Books, Inc.)

Coleman, Jill, (Caroline Jill)
    WaterYoga : water-assisted postures and stretches for
flexibility and well-being / by Jill Coleman. -- 1st ed.
    p. cm.
    Includes index

    1. Aquatic exercises. 2. Stretching exercises. 3. Yoga.
I. Title.
RA781.17.C65 1998   613.7'16
ISBN 0-9662970-0-8   QBI98-104

Published by Eglantine Press
10707 Sprinkle Lane, Owings MIlls, MD 21117
U.S.A.

Copyrighted material from the following books has been reprinted with permission from the following:

THE THINKING BODY, by Mabel E. Todd. Princeton Book Co.
ALEXANDER TECHNIQUE, THE JOY IN THE LIFE OF YOUR BODY, by Judith
    Stransky. Beaufort Books, Inc.

10 9 8 7 6 5 4 3 2 1

TABLE OF CONTENTS

ACKNOWLEDGEMENTS

I thank the following people alphabetically for their support as I developed WaterYoga. They are all A-PLUS and have my grateful recognition.

Steve Bonwit, licensed Physical Therapy Assistant. He was working at the Bennett Center for Health and Fitness at The New Children's Hospital in Baltimore, MD. during my last episodes of back spasms.

Dan Bowerman, massage and Reiki therapist.

Gloria Carpeneto, massage therapist. She is a Nationally Certified Massage Therapist and lecturer on adapting learning theory to the study of the body.

Cecelia Coleman, swimming coach in Baltimore, MD and Austin, TX. She said, "Of course you should write this book, Mom."

Cynthia Delafield, writer and long time exerciser with emphasis on yoga.

Bruce Kodish, Licensed Physical Therapist, Certified Alexander Technique teacher, and author.

Stephen Kilduff, advisor on organization of manuscript.

Florence Kuczynski, Electrical Engineer, advisor on physics.

Jim McFarland, Certified Massage Therapist and President of Muscle Therapy, Inc., swimming coach and analyst of body movement in competitive swimming.

Gloria McFarland, massage therapist in training.

Nancy Long and the formatting staff at Sir Speedy: Sidra Kirnon and Willie Sue Parker.

Eric McKeever, book author, publisher and dealer.

Giovanni Pescetto, acupuncturist, co-direct of the Baltimore Center for Wellness, a full facility of the Traditional Acupuncture Institute and faculty member of the Zero Balancing Association.

Kelly Russell, Feldenkrais instructor.

John Schumacher, Founder and Director of Unity Woods Yoga Studio, Bethesda, MD., Senior Certified Iyengar Teacher, member of the Certified International Yoga Teachers' Association.

Karlene Schwartz, biologist and faculty member, University of Massachusetts, Boston; author of science textbooks.

Peggy Taliaferro, participant in my first WaterYoga class.

Taronica Wilson, photographic assistant.

And I wish I could thank lots of people whose names I'll never know, who have seen me practicing WaterYoga and asked about it.

DISCLAIMER

Nothing in this book is intended to substitute for the advice of a trained health care professional. He or she can help you decide whether WaterYoga is appropriate for you, and guide you in proper practice habits. It is essential that you consult a medical professional or doctor of chiropractic for diagnosis and possible contraindications if you have or develop any adverse symptoms.

Although yoga as practiced in the Orient is perceived to have many medical applications, this book makes no claim for medical benefit from the practice of WaterYoga.

The publisher and author expressly disclaim any and all liability or responsibility to any person or entity for any injury, loss or harm of any kind, directly or indirectly, resulting from use of the postures and stretches and/or ideas and information contained in this book.

The information contained in this book is not held out to the reader as being complete. You are urged to read other available material. The author recommends material in the Sources section at the end of this book as a possible starting point. Nor is this book held out to the reader as being without mistakes, either typographical, substantive, or in manufacturing. In awareness of the possibility of there being such mistakes, a Suggestion Box page is included. You will find it on the reverse side of the Order Form at the very back of the book. Your thoughts, suggestions and criticisms are most welcome and will be incorporated into future editions as appropriate.

If you do not wish to be bound by this Disclaimer, you may return this book to the publisher for a full refund.

WATERYOGA

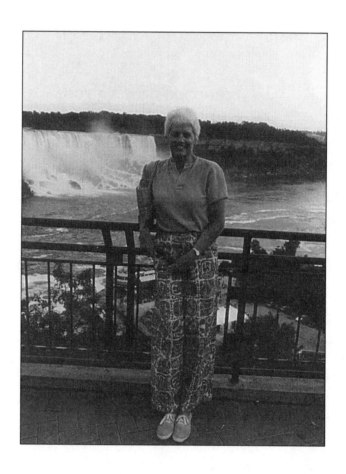

Photograph 1. Jill Coleman. This photograph introduces the author to you. Water is always welcome to her, but Niagara Falls is one place NOT to try WaterYoga.

Jill is an experienced competitive swimmer, diver, bicyclist, and runner. She is a graduate of Swarthmore College and the University of Maryland School of Law. She has three daughters and three grandchildren.

INTRODUCING WATER YOGA

Welcome to WaterYoga. WaterYoga offers you a unique approach to care of your bones and soft tissues, especially your back. It is a pleasant, non-demanding experience of salutary (healthy, wholesome) postures and stretches that you perform in warm water. Water makes your body feel weightless. So often the first comment I hear when I introduce someone new to WaterYoga is, simply, "A - a - a - h."

Perhaps the subtitle of WaterYoga should be just that:

"A - a - a - h. . . ."

WaterYoga unites two age-old wisdoms: the postures and stretches of yoga, and the warm water of the "baths" and "spas" of ancient Greece and Rome. Each enhances the effectiveness of the other.

WaterYoga is inherently suitable and productive for people of almost all ages and states of physical fitness. This is because, like yoga, it does not demand aggressive repetitions or require people of varying abilities to meet group norms. It is different from physical therapy, hydrotherapy, calisthenics, or aerobic exercise. Its essence is increasing flexibility, rather than strength.

WaterYoga induces relaxation and stretching of stiff, tight muscles, tendons and fasciae. As they relax and stretch, joints become more mobile. This is often accompanied by improvement in over-all physical well-being and heightened body awareness.

WaterYoga complements conventional medical treatment, which focuses on treatment of symptoms. For example, drugs often prescribed for arthritis pain include aspirin, ibuprofin, corticosteroids and non-steroidal anti-inflammatories such as Naprosyn. These drugs are effective for relief of pain, but do not address the underlying cause of pain. WaterYoga addresses the symptoms but also focuses on the physical conditions that precipitate the symptoms. It can be a non-toxic alternative to drug therapy and a non-invasive alternative to surgery.

If you are an experienced swimmer or athlete, or if you are already familiar with yoga, you may want to go directly to Part Four to read about the postures and stretches. If all this is brand new to you, however, you will probably want to read straight on before you get your feet wet. Or perhaps you will scan the Table of Contents to fill in the gaps in your understanding. If you want to read more deeply, explore the Glossary of Supplemental Information.

Even if you are a non-swimmer, you can practice WaterYoga. All you need is to feel comfortable standing in a few feet of water. As you become accustomed to practicing WaterYoga, your enjoyment of the water will increase.

In Part Four, see Sections I through II—Plus for WaterYoga Postures and Stretches in chest deep water. For shallow water and in the shower, see Section III. And if you are among the millions of people who are subject to back spasm, look especially at Part Five.

I encourage you to keep a record of your practice and your response to the postures and stretches. Parts Four and Five contain sample record pages which you are welcome to photocopy for continuing use.

And finally, I eagerly look forward to hearing from you about your own experience when you try WaterYoga. There is much to build on this foundation.

PART ONE: THE THEORY OF WATERYOGA

I. HOW AND WHY I DEVELOPED WATERYOGA

I came to develop WaterYoga in response to my own thirty years of experience with severe and intractable back pain and disability. After two operations (first a ruptured lumbar disc was removed, and two years later my lumbar spine was fused up through the third lumbar vertebra) and uncounted disabling back "episodes," I was offered the choice of further surgery, or "just live with it." During those thirty years I had learned that "living with it" meant losing a week out of my life, without warning, several times a year, disrupting every phase of my own life, and burdening my family, friends and co-workers.

Thirty years of protecting my unstable back against these periodic episodes of back spasm had left me increasingly inflexible. My back muscles were tight and rigid. Friends told me I sat and stood and walked as if I wore a body cast!

Three years ago, when I developed a painful, immobilizing kink in my right hip joint, my doctors talked about a hip operation. But, thinking about my rigid body, I wondered if this new hip problem might be a by-product of my back problem. When I thoroughly assessed my own body, I had to admit that I could no longer sit cross-legged on the floor. I could no longer touch my toes. I could not pick up my baby grandchild. Putting on panty-hose was often impossible. And I had had to give up tennis and running.

For exercise I went back to the competitive swimming that I had not done since college, and began to train regularly in the U.S. Masters swimming program. I began to attend an Iyengar yoga class. Yoga was a wonderful surprise! It was not sedentary, or new age meditation. It was strenuous, tiring, invigorating and restful all at the same time. On the yoga mat I realized how immobilized my hip joints actually were, although the doctors had found "normal range of motion" in them. After the yoga practice began to restore my hip flexibility I never had another kink. But my back was getting worse.

After the next back episode I visited an acupuncturist. He told me that the scar tissue from the two back operations seemed very tight and appeared to be anchored to the bones. These two scars down the middle of my back, from my coccyx to my waist, were fifteen years old. After the second operation I had worn a metal body brace for almost two years. This brace allowed virtually no movement of my spine or hip joints. Consider how these large surgical scars must have constricted during that time. Consider how, in the following years, the constricted scars must have limited my motion, especially forward and side bending. In addition, after thirty years of episodes of back spasm, my muscles must surely have shortened and lost flexibility.

With assistance from my acupuncturist, the scar tissue began to release its tightness. As the scar tissue released, I could start to work on lower back and hip flexibility in my yoga class. As my lower body became more flexible, my thoracic (upper) back responded as well. It, too, had become very tight, though I didn't realize it, in my absorption with the fragility of my lower back.

I believe that the scar tissue and adhesions in my back were released, at least partially, by acupuncture. So, in arguing for the benefits of WaterYoga I am glad to acknowledge the role of acupuncture in my story.

Despite my progress, a major episode occurred after only a few months. It put me in bed with all the major back muscles in spasm. I was unable even to sit up. All I had done was reach down to pick up a shoe. I could feel two protruding bones where my lower back should have been quite flat. My massage therapist made an emergency home visit. She saw the bony bumps that jutted out on either side of my spine and told me that they appeared to be part of the sacroiliac joints, and we agreed that massage was not appropriate for my distorted skeletal condition.

For several days my canvas corset, with its laces and belts pulled as tight as possible, held me stable. Even so, any false move in the bed could be treacherous. Just turning over took careful, sweaty minutes of exertion, using only my arms and legs to move the dead weight of my torso, knowing that any change in the bone/nerve relation in my spine could set off an excruciating spasm.

As the days of convalescence passed, I began to think about the therapy pool at the fitness center where I swam and trained when my back was well. I had used it occasionally to relax after a hard workout, and enjoyed its 90 degree water. My instincts told me that the warm water and weightlessness could help me.

I spent the next two weeks in bed. The bony bumps in my lower back were still there. When I tried to stand up my back was slumped over to the left and walking was perilous and exhausting. In the third week I finally recovered enough strength and balance to get down the stairs and into the car. I asked my daughter, Cecelia, to drive me to the therapy pool. I wore my corset over my bathing suit and walked like a mechanical toy through the weight room to the pool area, terrified that someone would bump into me and destroy my fragile balance. That short walk was a huge physical exertion that left me sweating.

"My god, what happened to you?" asked Steve, my trainer. He had shown me how to protect my back while riding a stationary bike and lifting weights.

"Bad back," was all I could whisper. I knew that the effort of forcing breath through my vocal chords to answer in a normal voice could trigger a spasm. He let me wear the corset into the pool.

This therapy pool is designed for people with all kinds of physical disabilities. It isn't very big, perhaps fifteen or twenty feet square. It has broad steps and a railing for walking down into and up out of the pool, and even a lifting chair on a sort of crane for lowering people into it and getting them back out again. The water is chest-deep. At first, it feels like a hot bath, but as the body acclimates, it feels just soothingly warm.

I eased myself down the steps, my body rigidly erect, my weight carefully supported by my arms as I held on to the railing. I was surprised that relief began to come even before the warm water reached my hips. Once in the middle of the pool, four feet deep, with my body supported by chest-deep water, I was not free of pain, but I was not in pain. I observed that I did not have to labor just to hold myself up. Steve brought me a plastic foam support called a "noodle," a wonderful invention that is described more fully later. I lay suspended upright in the water, my arms over the noodle to support my head, my feet dangling, toes barely touching the bottom, afraid to risk any movement that could disturb my back. Steve kindly told the other people in the pool how fragile I was. For an hour I lay suspended, doing nothing at all, thankful for my back's respite from pain, but also oddly able to identify the spastic grip of specific muscles because all my other muscles were so relaxed.

The next day I came back and stayed for two hours, for part of the time in a state somewhere between waking and sleeping. Or perhaps I reached a slightly altered state of consciousness, lulled by my weightlessness in the water, by its warmth and by my relief from pain.

On the third day, after half an hour in the warm water, my body seemed to suggest to me to sway from side to side very, very slowly, just an infinitesimal distance, as I lay suspended from my noodle. I visualized my spine slowly growing longer, and my sacroiliac joints separating enough to reseat themselves. I was disappointed that as I carefully climbed the steps out of the pool, my body weight began again to press down on my back. My posture was still distorted.

On the fourth day, after an hour in the therapy pool, my sacroiliac joints went back in place! I had a subtle sense of it when they shifted. Still in the water, I could feel that the bumps were gone. In addition, I could feel that the spasm had "let go." But I knew that the real test would come as I climbed the steps out of the pool.

When Cecelia came to take me home, the smile on my face told her that I was better. But we both knew that each step up those stairs meant more weight on my spine. When I reached the top the smile was still there. For the first time in three weeks I could stand up straight. The protrusions were still gone. I was still stiff and sore and vulnerable, but my body was no longer deformed!

Once my posture was normal, healing was very rapid. As always, the real proof of healing is the moment when the corset becomes an annoyance rather than a necessity. I took it off that same evening. The next day I was well enough to drive myself to the pool. As before, I lay for a while suspended from the noodle, but after fifteen minutes or so, I began to do some delicate swaying, first from side to side, then forward and back, like seaweed in a pond. What a treat! I cautiously widened the sidewise swaying. Within a week I felt completely healed.

After that I started some real stretching in the therapy pool. That felt so good that I systematically adapted my Iyengar yoga practice. It brought rapid progress in loosening both my hips and my back. I knew immediately that I could hold the stretches much longer in water than on the floor mat. I learned to feel specific muscles "let go."

When I reviewed my own history I realized that the combination of warm water and gentle stretching could be the key to health as well as healing. I began to call what I was doing "WaterYoga."

Today my back is stronger and more flexible and healthier than it has been in thirty years. My body no longer needs to be encased in a body cast made of my own muscles. The scar tissue from two back operations no longer pulls when I bend over. I am confident that WaterYoga has ended the cycle of episodes of back spasms. I no longer-consider surgery, either for my back or for my hip. I have incorporated WaterYoga into my life—two or three times a week. And especially at the first hint of tension in my back I hurry to the therapy pool.

In doing research for this book about WaterYoga, I looked deeply into various systems of postural training, most particularly the Alexander Technique and Feldenkrais. I realized that a very stiff neck sits on top of my now very limber back! A few neck stretches are beginning to loosen the cervical component of my spine. I feel the echo of this change everywhere and my body feels taller and lighter.

Out of my personal experience, and supportive consultation with many health care professionals, comes my book called WaterYoga. My advisors have suggested that I call myself an "independent scholar" because WaterYoga grows from my own thinking, analysis and innovation, rather than from any existing professional discipline.

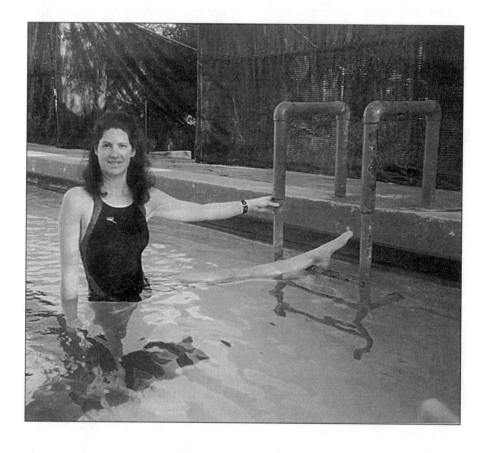

Photograph 2. Cecelia standing in Passive Side Leg Raise in hip deep water. She can intensify this stretch by flexing her ankle. If she can't reach the top step of the ladder, she can use a lower step.

II. WARM WATER

Warm water is wonderful for ailing and failing muscles. Simply being in warm water allows them to become softer, more relaxed, and less contracted. For many people water also has a calming, nurturing emotional effect.

In the western world, salutary (healthful) effects of warm water have been known since the golden age of the Greeks, who built pools at the locations of warm springs. "Taking the baths" was said to relieve rheumatism, gout, paralysis, neuralgia, internal complaints such as kidney stones and uric acid, sciatica, diseases of the liver, and "skin affections." Hippocrates, who is acknowledged today as the founder of western medicine used hydrotherapy.

Unfortunately, the history and popularity of thermal pools got lost at the fading of the Roman empire. Within the last decade, however, medical interest in warm water therapy has increased. Today, hospitals and fitness centers everywhere are installing therapy pools. Physicians are beginning to prescribe water therapy of varying sorts. These therapies are often covered by health insurance.

The mystical and religious power of water has also been recognized throughout history. The Greeks and Romans often dedicated their baths to the Gods. The Nile, in ancient Egypt, was said to be a continuation of the Milky Way, which was holy to the Egyptian priest-astronomers.

In the East, Hindus believe that the river Ganges is sacred to the goddess Ganga Ma. Its waters are said to flow from heaven through the hair of the goddess Shiva. The Hindu galaxy of gods intertwined with the Hindu theory of physical and spiritual health, which in ancient times was written down as the source of Ayurvedic medicine.

A water environment has four characteristics that are necessary in combination to make WaterYoga effective. They are its virtual equality to the weight of the human body, the hydrostatic pressure it exerts on the human body, its unique resistance to body movement, and its controllable temperature.

A. Weight

In water the human body is virtually weightless. That is, its mass weighs virtually the same as that of the mass of water it displaces. This is true in large part because the human body itself is typically about 70% water. When you "float," part of your body may be above the surface of the water and part below. The percentage of your body that stays above the water when you "float" is determined by the extent to which your body weighs less than water. If all of your body is below the surface, that means that your body weighs, cubic inch for cubic inch, more than water, and you will sink. Fortunately, most people float.

If you rest your upper arms on a float and let your torso, legs and feet dangle, your muscles and bones do not have to support the weight of your upper body and head. Your joints are not compressed. Your vertebrae can separate themselves a slight bit from each other, and your thighs (the bones are femurs) can separate a slight bit from your hip bones. The separation may be so subtle that you are not aware of it. You are actually doing a basic WaterYoga posture. I call it "Suspended Zen."

Weightless in water you can relax in a way that is impossible when you stand on the floor. As you stand erect on land, your bones are stacked one on top of the other, in a column. Each vertebra, each hip, each knee, each foot bears the weight of all the body mass above it. Even your neck must bear the weight of a head that may weigh more than fifteen pounds. Your muscles must be in a constant state of tension or "tone" to support this column. If not, your body would collapse.

Weightlessness in the water frees the body from the downward pressure of its own weight. For me, at least, relief comes because my vertebrae don't press against each other and my overworked muscles can rest. I can feel the pain dissipate. When the pain doesn't come back even after I have left the pool, I know that I have broken the cycle of nerve pain and muscle spasm that plagues so many back sufferers.

In addition, when you stand in neck-deep water you can push yourself off the bottom using just a toe or two, and rise effortlessly.

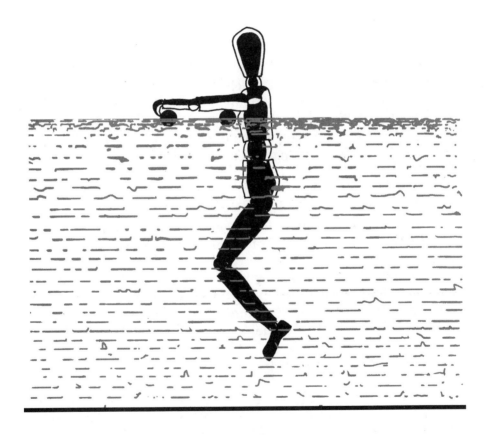

Illustration 1. Suspended Zen. This figure is the icon that I developed for illustrating WaterYoga, a generic person of no particular age sex size or shape. The posture called Zen, Suspended is a starting posture in which you pay special attention to the alignment of your back and pelvis as you go into a stretch. The two round discs show the placement of two simple flotation devices called "noodles."

Your feet softly touch the bottom again. You can't do that on a gym floor. In water you experience only the slightest impact.

B. Hydrostatic Pressure

A water environment exerts constant pressure on every surface of your body. This is called hydrostatic pressure. It works to keep your body in whatever position you assume. Thus, it enhances your ability to stay in the postures and stretches. You do not have this assistance in dry-land practice. (Hydrostatic pressure could be a problem during WaterYoga only if there is such severe lung disability or weakness in the chest muscles that it cannot be overcome during inhalation.)

C. Resistance

An important feature of WaterYoga is based on the unique resistance of water. Water offers a minimal but constant resistance to all movement in all directions. Although you must push a bit to move water, an easy push is enough. This means there is very little risk of straining a muscle while doing WaterYoga.

D. Warmth

In combination with these three characteristics of water, the true magic of WaterYoga is warm water. From earliest times, healthful springs with warm water were favored for "baths" and "spas." In warm water the muscles relax, allowing blood to flow freely throughout the body, nourishing the muscles, bones and other tissues. In contrast, the body reacts to cold water by causing the muscles and connective tissues to contract and become tense.

I conducted my first class in WaterYoga in a lovely outdoor pool. The trees around us and the sky above us were a tranquil backdrop. The water was about 80 degrees Fahrenheit, warm enough for teenagers to cavort in for hours, but it was too cold for the sustained quiet of WaterYoga. Within a few minutes some body temperatures were lowered to the blue-lipped, shivering stage. We learned that without cardiovascular exercise, we couldn't stay warm long enough to benefit from the postures or stretches.

I took my next class into a therapeutic pool, where the water was just over 90 degrees Fahrenheit. The difference was astounding. My students sensed the benefit of the warmth immediately. This was where I heard the first of many "A - a - a - h's." At the end of an hour, we were as warm and comfortable as when we first entered the water. A yoga teacher said, "I feel the letting go." This comment convinced us that warm water is essential for WaterYoga. (A writer in Yoga Journal notes that she had to combine yoga postures with strenuous martial arts movements in order to maintain body temperature.)

I also experienced the physiological response of my hands to warm water very vividly when I took a week-long class in felt-making. Felt is made by kneading wool fibers in warm soapy water. The fibers usually bond together ("full") after about fifteen minutes. After fulling my hands felt as if they had had a long and expert massage. Two members of our class had such severe arthritis in their hands that they had doubted that they could participate. Both commented that their hands felt much better at the end of the week! When I told this story to a body-worker friend, he said, without surprise, "Well, there is the power of warm water for you!"

We felt-makers also realized that physical relaxation and mental relaxation go hand in hand quite literally in felt-making. Felt-making was healing to minds and spirits as well as to arthritic fingers.

I have convinced myself during my three years of practicing WaterYoga that warm water is the optimum environment for lengthening tight muscles, opening constricted joints and increasing flexibility. It therefore increases the physical effectiveness of any yoga practice. I have found that as the warm water relaxes my body, it also relaxes my mind and soothes my spirit. This is beautifully consistent with the body/mind/spirit unity of yoga.

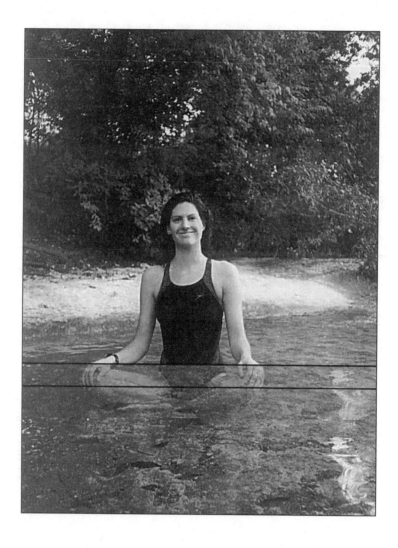

Photograph 3. Cecelia in Tailor's Seat A. Two horizontal lines show the general lower range of depth in which you can comfortably do this stretch. Cecelia is in an outdoor stream in beautiful natural surroundings. She could also do this stretch in a baby pool or on the seat of a hot tub or Jacuzzi.

III. YOGA

I have derived the Eastern component of WaterYoga from the postures and stretches of Iyengar Yoga. If you have been a practitioner, you will recognize many of them. WaterYoga has some characteristics in common with the "stretch classes" that are conducted at some fitness clubs, as well as with the warm-up stretches that athletes such as swimmers, runners and football players do. Its postural approach is consistent with Alexander Technique and Feldenkrais theories.

Yoga means "union" or "harmony" of the body and mind/spirit. The word "yoga" is derived from a Sanskrit word meaning yoke: the mind and body are designed to work together like two oxen that are yoked together. Yoga can be traced as far back as 4,000 B.C. in Asia and has been practiced continuously ever since. Yoga is not a religion, as some people assume from its association with Taoism and Buddhism. It is not associated with any supernatural power of any kind.

Since the 1950s, yoga has become better understood and more popular in the United States. Several schools of yoga have developed. These include Hatha and Iyengar, among others. My experience has been with Iyengar yoga, which is considered to be more physically strenuous than many. Though the various schools of yoga differ somewhat in practice, they all share the principle of harmony of body and mind/spirit. If one accepts that the body, the mind and the spirit are integral and interlaced, then health—body health—is the physical aspect of the health of all three. Body-wisdom, or awareness, is the sense of unity and involvement of mind and spirit with the body.

The practice of yoga consists of assuming and holding gentle stretches and postures, or "poses." Breathing is an important part of proper yoga practice. So is an atmosphere of quiet and harmony, which induces self-awareness. Properly done, yoga increases strength, endurance, and balance; encourages proper posture, improves vascular, heart, and lung function, and facilitates relaxation. Yoga also increases flexibility by lengthening and conditioning the muscles and connective tissues. This increases range of motion in the joints and opens up the joint spaces to minimize abrasive movement of the bones against each other. Yoga stimulates circulation of blood and lymph to cleanse, nourish and energize the organs and tissues, and bring oxygen to the cells. It provides healthful massage to the internal organs, increasing their vitality and functioning power. It is also thought to stimulate circulation of the life energy which many cultures call "Ch'i."

Yoga may also help in managing daily stress and release the muscular tension that often causes headaches, stiff necks and backaches.

Many people, in the course of the physical practice of yoga, perceive spiritual and mental benefits as well.

Yoga postures and stretches are precise and astonishingly complex. You will enhance your practice of WaterYoga if you practice conventional yoga or read about it.

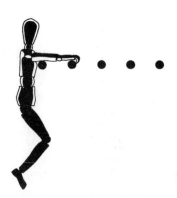

IV. PEOPLE WHO BENEFIT FROM WATERYOGA

WaterYoga offers benefits to men and women of all ages and wide levels of conditioning, from the most vigorously trained athlete to the totally sedentary. As a general rule, I believe that WaterYoga encourages the body's inherent desire to be healthy and to heal itself.

• **Postural Problems**. WaterYoga can help people who have postural problems such as forward head, rounded shoulders, slouch, collapsed chest, sway back (lordosis) and arthritis, and even the postural aspects of scoliosis. (It has not yet been determined whether any activity in water is useful as protection against osteoporosis. I am glad that the subject is being investigated. In any event, people with postural problems linked to osteoporosis may find at least temporary postural relief.)

As far back as 1937, Mabel E. Todd argued that the human body is subject to all the laws of physics that operate on architectural structures, the most influential being gravity. She traced many postural problems to failure to stack the heavy body components — the head, thorax and pelvic bowl — on the central gravitational axis of the body,

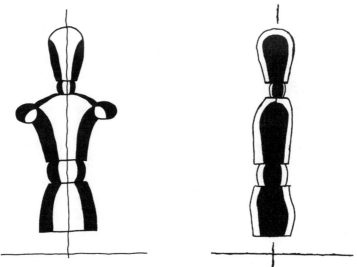

Illustration 2. Gravitational axis of the body: front and side views of stack of head, thorax and pelvis.

and failure to balance the compression of the spine with upward pull of the abdominal muscles in supporting the side-loaded thorax and the braced pelvis, both of which hang forward of the spine. She argued that because many musculoskeletal problems arise from poor posture, correcting poor posture may alleviate, or prevent orthopedic problems.

A thirty year old woman with whom I swim has a slight lateral curvature of her upper spine. It is not enough to be labeled scoliosis. I can see that one shoulder is slightly higher than the other, but the spinal curvature only becomes evident when she bends forward. She told me that perhaps a third of women have this curvature. I see, among my

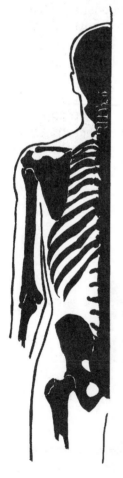

friends who are in their sixties, an accentuation of this kind of curvature. She plans to start a WaterYoga program to increase flexibility in her spine and relax and re-educate her shoulder and back muscles. I hope her back will be straight when she is in her sixties.

I know that pressure on one specific point along my thoracic spine echoes in one of my upper left molars. My massage therapist and I tested it for most of one session. Another friend suffers from tension in her neck and migraine headaches. I wonder if her neck pain is an echo of the imbalance in her back. I wonder if her migraine headache is an echo of her spinal imbalance.

Many forms of posture and movement education are adaptable to WaterYoga. For example, the Alexander Technique was developed by an Australian actor, F. Matthias Alexander (1869 - 1955). In the Alexander Technique, one notices one's undesirable posture and movement patterns and learns to replace them with healthful postures and movements. Feldenkrais movements are based on a similar theory, but are more active. I have included a long section on posture in the

Illustration 3. Gravitational axis of the body: half of the skeleton viewed from behind

Glossary of Supplemental Information. Understanding the physics of posture under the influence of gravity clarifies the benefits of improving posture in the weightless environment of warm water.

If surgery has corrected posturally induced problems, WaterYoga can facilitate improvement of posture and movement. If the posture is corrected, the problems may be less likely to recur.

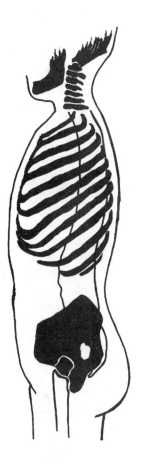

• **Post-Surgical Recovery.** Patients who are recovering from surgery, especially orthopedic surgery, can begin to regain range of motion and muscle tone in a weightless water environment sooner than in land-based therapy. For instance, they may have insufficient strength to perform post-surgical exercises, but in the weightless water environment they can begin to tone muscles and stretch joints without effort or risk to unhealed soft tissue and bones. WaterYoga can often be commenced as soon as incisions are healed, long before the discomfort of land-based exercises can be tolerated.

Illustration 4. Side view of skeleton in good alignment.

• **Post-Surgical Scarring.** WaterYoga is an important tool for preventing the ill effects of post-surgical scarring. Mary Pullig Schatz, M.D., discusses the nature and treatment of scar tissue very clearly in BACK CARE BASICS, A DOCTOR'S GENTLE YOGA PROGRAM FOR BACK AND NECK PAIN RELIEF.

The body heals itself by producing scar tissue, which is good, but scar tissue may develop harmful characteristics. For instance, over time, even after as little as six months or less, scar tissue begins to lose elasticity and becomes resistant to stretching. Recent scars can be kept elastic through body movement.

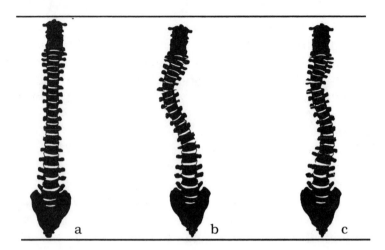

Illustration 5. Three back views of the spine. The thoracic and lumbar vertebrae are shown in black and the discs in white. The cervical (neck) vertebrae and the sacrum/coccyx are shown in black. View a is a normal spine. The spines in views b and c are deformed by scoliosis in the classic "C" and "S" curves.

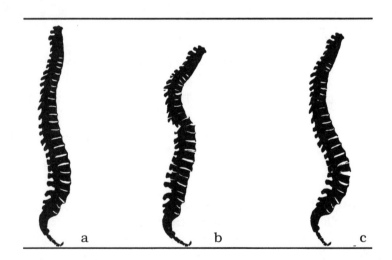

Illustration 6. Three side views of the spine. The thoracic and lumbar vertebrae are shown in black and discs in white. The cervical (neck) vertebrae and the sacrum/coccyx are shown in black. View a is a normal spine. The spines in views b and c are deformed by humping and by lordosis.

Tissue that has been scarred and traumatized also tends to shrink and pull together, putting damaging stress on neighboring bones and tissue and limiting range of motion. A nerve in a scarred area can become entrapped in scar tissue, causing pain. WaterYoga is a valuable preventive for nerve damage caused by constriction of surrounding tissue or by entrapment.

With patience, even old scars can be induced to stretch and lengthen in WaterYoga.

Adhesions often develop from scar tissue. Adhesions are superfluous or exaggerated fibrous connections to other tissue, bones, and even nerves. They can severely limit motion, and put damaging strain on adjoining tissues. Adhesions can be prevented by keeping the surgical site supple following surgery. Sometimes existing adhesions can be released through stretching, movement and massage.

• **Back Spasm.** Sudden episodes of excruciating and incapacitating back pain are a common complaint in men and women of all ages. WaterYoga devotes a special section to the care of back spasm. See Part Five.

In the acute phase of such a back episode, performing any postures and stretches is unthinkable, as any sufferer knows, but the soothing warmth of water and its weightlessness can bring temporary relief. During the healing phase, gentle stretches encourage the muscles to relax. During the rehabilitation phase, posture can be improved, muscles strengthened and flexibility and elasticity increased.

• **Disc Disease.** The discs are intervertebral pads composed of a fibrous outer layer and a gelatinous filling. In the normal back, the intervertebral discs are nourished by fluids and gases which diffuse through the disc spaces. They are not, like the rest of the body, directly nourished by the blood stream. A healthy spine expands by as much as an inch overnight when the vertebra separate from each other, while the body is lying down and the vertical pressure of standing is eliminated. This nightly separation of the vertebrae allows the discs to expand and be nourished.

When the weight of the upper body compresses the vertebrae, the upper and lower surfaces of the discs are temporarily sealed off from nourishment. For optimum disc health, it seems that periods of both compression and decompression are necessary. This is achieved in the day/night cycle, through movement of the spine, and through exercise. A disc that is unrelievedly compressed by spasm or by too much weight or by stiffness, however, cannot expand to receive nourishment. Furthermore, an injured disc does not heal as well as muscles and bones, since it is not directly nourished by blood.

Weightlessness during WaterYoga temporarily restores an environment in which the discs can be nourished. Nourishment is enhanced by gentle constant movement of the spine. Postures and stretches in which you hang vertically from a noodle are especially helpful for this kind of movement of the spine.

• **Back Problems.** Many back pain sufferers are frustrated that doctors have little to offer as a remedy for back problems. Yet back problems are among the most common ailments in America and perhaps the least helped by standard, or allopathic, medicine. Dr. Hans Kraus,

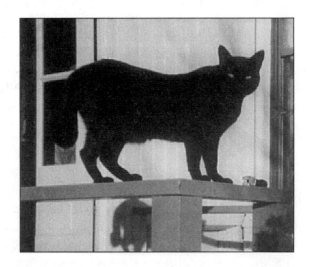

Photograph 4. Cat. See how easily the spine is slung between the supporting columns of the front and rear legs.

the physician who helped President Kennedy with his back problem, has claimed that muscle spasm and muscle tension, together with the whole syndrome of neck, back, and leg pains, are due basically to poor posture. Correct your posture and postural habits, he has said, and the problems will not occur. Postural habits include activities we perform daily, even talking on the telephone.

Because the human spine is vertical, it is uniquely subject to the compressive pressures of gravity and weight. We humans must deal all our lives with the ills caused by compression and distortion of the spine. Just think of a cat to understand the advantage of the horizontal spine. Its organs hang like clothes on a clothesline, not heaped on top of each other against a vertical spine. Its weight transfers to four feet instead of two.

The fundamental principles of correct human body posture are addressed by teachings as disparately generated as those of the ancient yoga masters, and in modern times by F. Matthias Alexander, Moshe Feldenkrais, Mabel E. Todd, and Ida Rolf, as well as the great modern yoga master, B. K. S. Iyengar. I find a marvelous consistency among them all in adapting their principles to WaterYoga.

• **Low (Lumbar) Back Nerve Pain.** Low back pain can occur when a nerve is pinched between the adjacent vertebrae. It can trigger referred pain down the leg as far as the foot. It can also cause numbness and even paralysis in the leg. Causes include narrowing of the disc space, protrusion of the disc into the spinal canal (herniation), rupture or disintegration of the disc, arthritis, and even postural problems. The weightless environment and gentle stretching of WaterYoga open up the spaces between the vertebrae, temporarily relieving pressure on the nerves.

• **Sacroiliac Pain.** In the lower spine there are joints on either side of the sacrum where it meets the pelvic bones. These joints can become displaced. Even slight displacement can bring on a cycle of inflammation, pain and muscle spasm. As with spasm in the low back, the absence of weight-caused skeletal compression and the warm water invite the sacroiliac joints to re-seat themselves properly.

• **Arthritis.** Arthritis describes a variety of joint symptoms including pain, swelling and limitation of movement. It affects tens of millions of people in the United States. Traditionally, exercising arthritic joints was not recommended for fear of damaging the affected joints, but present thinking embraces exercise to increase range of motion and flexibility, and to build strength in the muscles around the joints. The Arthritis Foundation and the YMCA of America have developed water exercise programs especially for arthritis therapy.

WaterYoga provides a different but compatible approach to the management of arthritis. Weightlessness and the moist heat of a warm pool in themselves form an environment that eases pain. Gentle WaterYoga stretches are effective in increasing flexibility and increasing range of motion without pain and without the jolts of impact on a hard floor. If the arthritic condition limits walking and land-based exercise, joint movement plus some muscle conditioning is often possible in the weightless environment of water.

• **Disabilities.** Congenital deformities, strokes and degenerative diseases are among the many physical problems that limit children as well as adults in their movement. Most therapeutic pools are equipped with easy steps and guard rails for easy entry and exit. Some have wheelchair access into the water.

A massage therapist asked me whether I was ready to recommend WaterYoga to the wheelchair-bound. I have not personally explored that possibility, and do not have the medical experience to say yea or nay, but I have often seen wheelchairs, and other prostheses as well, parked at the edge of the therapy pool that I use. I believe that WaterYoga should be explored for its potential as an addition to the growing variety of activities for handicapped and disabled persons. Therapeutic pools may also offer a safe environment for blind persons.

• **Well-Body Care.** No matter how fit you are, if you overwork your body you will find WaterYoga to be an effective muscle loosener. WaterYoga eases sore muscles, tightness and strain after extraordinary physical activity, such as too much yard work or tennis. Serious athletes can relieve stiff, overworked muscles after training or competition. The gentle stretches of WaterYoga also help to dissipate lactic acid, which is the metabolic waste product that accumulates in the tissues during strenuous exercise. Athletes are cautioned, however, that WaterYoga will not increase muscle mass or strength.

Post-exercise soreness can be evidence of muscle inflammation. It can cause muscles to contract, which means decreased range of motion. Gentle stretches, rather than more muscle-stressing activity, is increasingly recognized as the best way to counteract muscle soreness.

Fixed posture or immobility that results from protracted sedentary activity can also lead to stiffness and muscle tension. Sitting at a computer or telephone and while driving are known culprits, especially as they affect the shoulders and neck. A half-hour of WaterYoga is helpful in relieving this stiffness and muscle tension.

WaterYoga may be "just what the doctor ordered" for minor back problems. The absence of weight (downward pressure) allows your spine to decompress (vertebrae to separate slightly from each other) as you develop flexibility and tone your back and abdominal muscles in a safe environment.

• **Men.** After reading an article in the Yoga Journal (May/June 1995) called "Real Men Do Yoga," I realized that I must point out that men as a special group can benefit from WaterYoga. The author states that only about a fourth of yoga practitioners are men. After skeptically joining a yoga class, he got results such as learning how to relax and dissolving accumulated stress that he had unknowingly held in his body for years. Within months, his weight and blood pressure dropped. I think even professional football players will be pleasantly surprised by WaterYoga.

• **Obesity.** The obese person, relieved of the burden of his or her own weight, can perform the postures and stretches of WaterYoga on equal terms with the thinnest neighbor.

• **Aging.** Older bodies tend to stiffen. This is partly because collagen, a prime component of connective tissue, tends to lose its extensibility (pseudo-elasticity) in the aging process. Reduced range of motion can occur anywhere in the body: back, hips, knees, hands, shoulders and neck. The stretches and postures of WaterYoga loosen stiff joints and muscles to preserve and even increase range of joint motion.

In addition, older bodies tend to slump and to shrink. At 67, I am at the age when this happens. I have been doing floor-based yoga and swimming for six years, and WaterYoga for three years during the crucial time when we notice the onset of slumping and shrinking. Is it just coincidence that I am now taller than friends who used to be taller than I? Or are stretching and attention to posture part of the key to height retention as we get older?

• **Stress.** People who are battling stress find warm water physically relaxing. Many relaxation techniques to reduce physical stress that are performed "on land" are actually more effective in warm water. Indeed, some people find complete physical relaxation more attainable when the body is supported by water than when lying down.

Emotional stress reveals itself by fast pulse, fast shallow breathing, tightness in the throat, clenching of the jaw, and a sick feeling in the stomach, as well as tense muscles. Many good books are available which address the mental stress that accompanies, causes, interacts with and/or intensifies physical stress, and describe stress reduction techniques that are adaptable to water.

• **Pregnancy.** WaterYoga can be a special treat to pregnant women. A pregnant woman carries an unbalanced load of as much as forty or fifty pounds during her last trimester of pregnancy. After she has carried that load all day, imagine her joy at putting it down for an hour. That is what happens when she submerges her body in water: she and her baby become weightless.

In the late months of pregnancy, a pregnant woman's posture can be seriously distorted by the unbalanced load. In the warm pool, her posture can return to normal, relieving strain on joints and supporting tissues. And metaphorically as well as actually, she enters the very environment that she provides for her developing baby.

WaterYoga can be adapted to exercises for childbirth preparation. Pregnant women should, of course, seek medical approval and advice before practicing WaterYoga. They should also be aware that water that is too warm could be dangerous for mother and child.

PART TWO: STARTING WATERYOGA

I. BEFORE YOU GET YOUR FEET WET

You can practice WaterYoga in a class, if one is available; or alone where there is a lifeguard, or with a buddy. The buddy system is a safety requirement for swimming. A buddy can also be a "coach" to observe you in postures and stretches.

Better yet, try to find a suitable teacher. I strongly recommend this because a teacher can help you learn to do the postures correctly. Learning any physical activity from books or even tapes can lead to errors in form or even physical harm. As a springboard diver, I would never have considered practicing without my teacher present. Diving calls for the same kind of subtle precision that is vital to Yoga. It is also similar to WaterYoga when the body lies weightless and unattached at the apex of each dive.

If you have prior experience in yoga you will find it easy to adapt it to WaterYoga.

If you have had no prior experience with yoga, however, you will want to find a good book to augment your understanding of yoga postures and principles. Like floor-based yoga, WaterYoga invites total mind and body absorption. As you become more aware of your body structure, and in the water medium you can often articulate your own muscle structure more easily than on land, you will find the process intensely interesting. You will not be bored.

If you join a WaterYoga class, remember that, just as you must always respect the teacher, you always deserve the teacher's respect. This means that you should do only what your own body tells you is appropriate for you. Don't do what your body tells you is inappropriate even if you see the rest of the class doing it easily or even if your teacher insists. Explain your limitations before the class begins or as soon as you realize you may get into trouble in a posture or stretch. If you have a physical problem, you and your health care professional together should select the postures and stretches that are appropriate for your own special needs.

Balance your class environment with the knowledge that your practice of yoga is internal to you, and in that sense, is a solitary and independent self-exploration. Have a firm pact with your body that you will do WaterYoga at your own pace, frequency and intensity, and respect your own tolerance for stretching. Since in WaterYoga nobody else touches you, or manipulates your body, nobody else can strain or hurt you. (The exception might be a disabled person who would need the physical support of a therapist to maintain balance and security in the pool.)

If you are new to the water environment you haven't realized yet that it's hard to push yourself to the point of strain or harm in water. This statement is not meant to be taken as permission to persevere through pain. Some kinds of pain are "acceptable" but others are warnings to stop. Be sure to read and understand the section on pain if you are not familiar with the difference between true pain and "good hurt."

Here are questions I am frequently asked about WaterYoga:

• "How many times a week must I do this?" The answer is, "About as frequently or as seldom as you feel the need or benefit."

• "How many repetitions must I do?" WaterYoga doesn't work in terms of repetitions. The benefit comes from holding a posture or stretch. The duration is generally around 30 seconds. But sometimes you will want to hold a posture for minutes or more.

• "When will I see results?" There is no universal answer. Benefits can come quickly but long-term value is perceived slowly, after long practice.

Bones and muscles of the human anatomy interact with beautiful precision to form posture and create movement. Good posture and efficient movement are not arbitrarily called "good" and "efficient." There is a rationale behind them. For people who ask what that rationale is, I have included sections on physics and human anatomy in the Glossary of Additional Information. They help to explain the "why's" of the postures and stretches.

A final reminder as to the right frame of mind for WaterYoga: don't compete, either with yourself or with others. You are not in a group you have to out-perform, or even try to "keep up with." Like the trip of a thousand miles, you are going to "start with a single step," as you slowly and gently introduce your body to proper skeletal alignment.

Each time you practice WaterYoga you will build on all the preceding practices, slowly and cumulatively. There is no goal, no completion, no perfection at the end of training. There is no score-card or final exam. Nobody will be better than you and nobody will be worse than you. Avoid measuring your results against your own expectations, or against the achievements of others. Don't dwell on goals or failures. These are not in the vocabulary of yoga.

I wish you a good experience.

II. WHAT WATERYOGA IS NOT.

This brief section clarifies what WaterYoga is not. It is not "New Age," or hippie, or cult-based, or based on physical contortions and drone-like chanting while in an altered state of mind.

WaterYoga is not a medical treatment. It is not (not yet, at least) a form of physical therapy. It is not, strictly speaking, even exercise. It has no aerobic effect. It does not build muscle mass or strength or enhance endurance. It does not promise weight loss.

WaterYoga is not a competitive event.

And finally, WaterYoga is not a religion. It is not Hindu, or Buddhist, or Taoist, or Zen, any more than it is Catholic, or Jewish or Protestant or Quaker. Practitioners of yoga may follow any of these religions, or none of them.

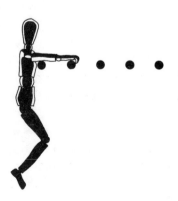

III. PHRASES FOR WATERYOGA PRACTICE

In WaterYoga, as in conventional yoga, several phrases are significant. You will see them often as the postures and stretches are described. One or two may have already sneaked into this text.

• You **"practice"** WaterYoga in the sense of practicing medicine or law, not in the sense of memorizing a speech to deliver once and forget, or learning to type. You practice WaterYoga in the archaic sense of the word: to carry on or to engage in a process. The Greek root is most descriptive: you "experience." You are a practitioner.

• As practitioner, you **"go into"** a posture. There is a subtle but important difference between "going into" a posture and "assuming" a posture. Going into conveys the idea of an ongoing process, not a single completed action.

• When you **"activate"** a part of your body you use (tense) certain muscles in that part of the body.

• You **"open up"** a joint by visualizing the space between the bones. This allows you to "go more deeply" into the posture.

• You **"image"** a joint, or a set of muscles, or even a mental process during a stretch or posture, by creating a picture of yourself in it—visualizing it. This helps your body to understand what is expected of it. Your mind teaches your body. Imaging can be very specific, or it can be general. You can also image yourself receiving and welcoming its benefits. In some indescribable way, you seem to set up a dialogue between your mind and your body,

• **"Holding"** a stretch means staying in it long enough for the connective tissue to respond. This involves almost no physical movement. Holding does not mean struggling or forcing. Physiologically, the connective tissues normally respond within about thirty seconds. During this time, you observe your physical body and perhaps your mental response to the posture. In WaterYoga, holding a posture is much easier than it is on land, so you may comfortably hold a posture a minute or more. Spastic muscles may ask you for many minutes.

• **"Breathing into"** joints, tissues or organs means directing an image of your breath into them. Although "breathing into" is a state of mind, remember that the mind and body are joined ("yoked") in Yoga.

• **"Inviting"** a muscle or ligament to "let go" is a conscious alternative to breathing into it. An invitation is never insistent or commanding. Don't force. Hold the stretch a little longer, if your body has accepted the invitation to let go.

• **"Letting go"** is the lengthening response of the body to a posture or stretch. An experienced practitioner actually senses the stretching, relaxing or lengthening. The "letting go" is a signal to "go more deeply" into the posture or stretch. Some practitioners feel that a muscle or tendon or ligament itself senses the intent of the mind.

• **"Going more deeply"** means slowly intensifying a posture or stretch, in response to the "letting go" in careful awareness of the good feeling of the stretch, stopping short of the bad feeling of pain or strain.

• **"Imprint"** is the new feeling in your muscles and connective tissues in response to a postural change or a letting go. An imprint may stay with you after you leave the water. If so, your body is learning something important.

• **"Emptying the mind"** means nothing more than turning your thoughts inward, away from the outside world. Your mind is empty when it contains only your breathing and your body in the posture or stretch. Only the empty mind is the receptive mind. The idea of "empty mind" comes from the Eastern practice of Zen.

• **"Soft eyes"** helps you to go into the posture and to empty your mind. Yoga instructors use this phrase to describe an open-eyed, unfocused gaze into the space above the floor a few feet in front of you, or into nothing. Soft eyes is the opposite of "hard eyes," which means staring, squinting, trying to see clearly.

IV. FACILITIES FOR WATERYOGA

All you need for WaterYoga practice is water that is (a) warm, (b) quiet and (c) of sufficient depth to accommodate your postures and stretches.

As said before, warm water is absolutely crucial. WaterYoga is not for the Polar Bear Club. **Make sure the water is not so cold that your muscles might contract.** Make sure you can *stay* warm for a substantial period of time. A leisurely WaterYoga practice may take an hour or more.

At the other extreme, make sure that the water is not too warm. Some people can stand only fifteen or twenty minutes. It's a highly individual thing. I have stayed in a warm pool as long as three hours and wished that I could stay longer, but I am not bothered by heat. Pregnant women, and people with high blood pressure, heart problems, strokes, and neurological disorders must get advice and approval from a medical advisor. Some elderly people might find warm water enervating.

• **Therapeutic pools.** Heated pools known as "therapeutic pools" are perfectly suited for WaterYoga. They are typically about four to five feet deep. They are designed to be sufficiently deep that almost all adults can stand comfortably chest deep in them while retaining secure footing on the bottom. The water will feel HOT at first, but your body soon adjusts and welcomes the soothing warmth. It's pretty well impossible to get chilled in water that may be as hot as 90 degrees. Many therapeutic pools use chemicals such as calcium hypochlorite that are less harsh than old-fashioned chlorine, or use alternatives to chemo-bactericides.

Many therapeutic pools are built as part of medical facilities. As an extension of hydrotherapy, their salutary effect is rapidly becoming well known. Fitness centers are beginning to include them. And almost all first-class retirement facilities are building them and featuring them in their promotional materials.

With increasing use of therapy pools for non-medical reasons, the name "therapeutic pool" may have become too narrow. Because "therapy" implies some kind of disease that needs curing some healthy people may be put off when I suggest WaterYoga in the therapy pool. On the other hand, insurance can in some cases cover "therapy" in a therapy pool. This is a significant financial factor that is worth checking into with your medical insurance provider.

• **Lakes, beaches, pools.** A lake or a beach is fine for WaterYoga, if the depth and temperature are right and the water is quiet. Of course, tolerance for cold water is a factor. Outdoor air temperature is also a factor. If you get cold as soon as you get out, you will put all your newly found relaxation at risk.

Any swimming pool, indoor or outdoor, public or private, is fine if it is warm enough and not too crowded.

Even the IRS has been convinced of the healing effect of swimming so you may get a tax break for building your own pool if your doctor prescribes swimming and if there is no other convenient facility. Consult your tax advisor as well as your architect.

Many postures and movements are effective in water too deep to stand in, and others are ideal in water that is only a few inches deep. I enjoy exploring the possibilities of WaterYoga under water, in the deep end of a pool or fifteen feet down in a lake. Down that deep the slight increase in pressure makes the body a little leaner.

Salt water is slightly more buoyant than plain water. You will feel that your body rides a little higher in salt water. And you may have to accommodate some postures to your added buoyancy. I experimented in the warm salt water bay of Montevideo, Uruguay, in December of 1966 (summer in the southern hemisphere), and found some postures and stretches easy to do without a flotation support. Some standing-in-shoulder-deep-water postures, on the other hand, were impossible because my feet kept drifting up off the bottom. The key is to innovate.

• **Whirlpools, hot tubs, Jacuzzis.** A whirlpool, hot tub or Jacuzzi may be used for some postures and stretches if the water temperature, depth and area are right and you turn off the jet mechanism so that the water agitation does not disturb your balance or detract from your body awareness.

• **"Endless Pool."** The "Endless Pool" may be adapted to WaterYoga by disarming the current-producing mechanism and raising the water temperature to 90 degrees. Endless Pools are small (8' by 15') and can be installed outside or inside for home use. They are designed to provide a resistance current against which a swimmer simulates distance swimming. The depth of an Endless Pool, 3 1/2 feet, may be a limiting factor.

• **Bathtub, baby pool.** Your bathtub will provide room for one or two shallow-water stretches. A child's wading pool can be used for sitting and reclining postures and stretches.

• **Shower!** Although your bathroom shower is not by any means a "pool," a gentle stream of warm water will enhance stretches of your neck, shoulders, back, hands and feet.

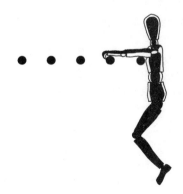

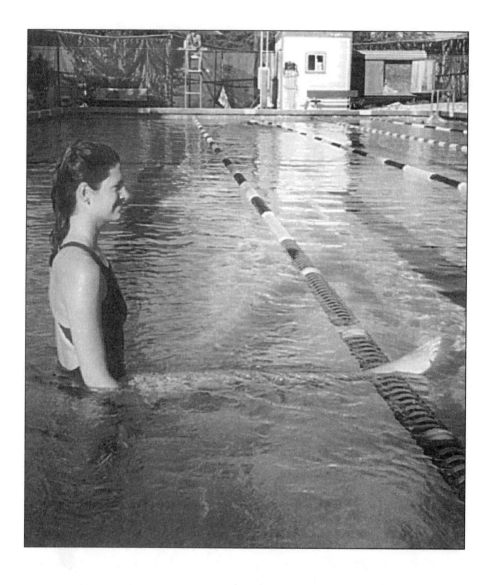

Photograph 5. Cecelia in Passive Straight Leg Raise. She is supporting herself on the lane rope, standing on the bottom of the pool. She can intensify this stretch by flexing her ankle and by lifting her sternum. She is so steady on her feet that she does not need a noodle.

V. EQUIPMENT FOR WATERYOGA

You need very little equipment for WaterYoga.

• **"Noodle."** A "noodle" is the only piece of equipment that is absolutely necessary for WaterYoga. A noodle is a flexible plastic foam cylinder about 3 inches in diameter and about five feet long. It provides just enough flotation to keep your head and shoulders above water when your feet are free of the bottom. Most pools have them on hand. Toy stores and even grocery stores sell them.

As I experimented with my noodle, I discovered that if one noodle is good, two are even better for many of the postures and stretches. I use one for flotation and the other for stabilization. I think that the second noodle will be a great comfort to people who are not totally secure in the water.

Therapy pools often provide plastic foam "belts" for flotation during "aqua-jogging." I tried one but found it bad for WaterYoga for two reasons. First, it does not relieve downward gravitational upper body pressure on the back. You are not weightlessly suspended in a belt. Second, your body is not stabilized in a vertical position. This means that you must constantly be muscularly and mentally involved in keeping yourself upright. Extra work to maintain erect posture may cause harmful strain to back muscles while doing WaterYoga. My own experience was that I was unable to relax while wearing the flotation belt. For a third of the price, the noodle is better flotation equipment.

• **Water bottle.** Bring a water bottle! Your body dehydrates in water, even though you may not realize it. Weigh yourself before and after an hour of WaterYoga. Each pound you lose is a pint of water that you should replace during your practice, not after.

• **Bathing suit.** By all means wear a light-weight body-fitting suit. You do not want to continually feel the drag of cloth flapping around your body. Do not let vanity, modesty, embarrassment or convention keep you in a dress-maker suit or "trunks." I promise that once you experience the freedom of a tank suit, you will never enjoy an old-fashioned suit as much again. You will also be very pleased to find that it dries overnight.

In WaterYoga you need never put your head under water. But you may find some of the following swimming aids useful.

• **Bathing Cap.** A bathing cap is not necessary, but it protects your hair from splashes.

• **Goggles, Face Mask.** Goggles or face mask allow you to see as well under water as you do in air and they protect your eyes from disinfectant that pools must use.

• **Ear-Plugs.** Ear-plugs will help to protect against ear infections. Many swimmers use ear drops made of equal parts of water, white vinegar and distilled alcohol used before and after swimming to prevent, and even cure, "swimmer's ear."

• **Nose-Clips.** Occasionally, someone finds nose-clips helpful, but try to get along without them if you can because they prevent you from breathing naturally.

• **Waterproof Shoes.** Some people like to wear waterproof shoes in the pool. I prefer the feeling of being barefooted, and I'm willing to risk getting athlete's foot. Most sporting goods stores carry bathing shoes.

• **Sunscreen.** If you are outside, make it waterproof, of course.

• **Zippered plastic bag**. Take this book with you to waterside in a clear waterproof bag to refresh your understanding of postures and stretches.

I personally do not like snorkels. For me a snorkle is nothing more than an unnecessary complication. But it allows you to breathe with your face under water. If you are more comfortable with it, by all means give it a try.

VI. RULES FOR WATERYOGA

The following rules are simple common sense. And before you start WaterYoga, reread the disclaimers at the beginning of this book.

1. MEDICAL RULES: Always obey these medical rules.

• **Get a physical checkup before you start.** Show your doctor this book. He or she may want to read it if not familiar with yoga or the principles of hydrotherapy. Explain where you will be practicing WaterYoga. Discuss the water temperature. This is especially important if you have heart disease, high blood pressure or circulatory problems, if you have had a stroke, if you are pregnant, or if you are older. ("Older," of course, is a relative and highly personal evaluation. The important thing is to use good judgment about your capabilities, no matter what your age.) Discuss any physical problems that might impact on your practice of WaterYoga.

• **Do not substitute WaterYoga for, or use it to override, prescribed medical treatment.** If you are under medical supervision, make sure that your doctor assures him- or herself that WaterYoga is compatible with your medical treatment and/or physical therapy.

• **Be alert to pain.** If existing pain becomes more severe, or if headache, fever, vomiting, or loss of bladder or bowel control develops in association with back pain, or if you develop numbness or weakness in your arm(s) or leg(s), consult your doctor immediately. Read the section on pain in Part Three.

2. RULES FOR USING A POOL. These are hard and fast rules, as well as common sense. Although they seem obvious, every one of them is violated.

• **Never go into the water alone.** Just as you must never swim alone, you should never practice WaterYoga alone. If there is a lifeguard, tell him or her what you are doing. Alert him or her to any injury or physical condition that might become a problem. If there is no lifeguard, find someone to go with you. You must use the buddy system: each of you is responsible for the safety of the other.

• **Don't go in a pool if you have an infection or communicable disease.** The warm damp air around a pool is a fertile breeding ground for germs and bacteria (e.g. athlete's foot) which you could pass on to others. If you feel vulnerable to "catching" something from others, use sensible judgment as to whether to stay away until your resistance improves.

• **Respect other persons who are sharing the water with you.** Take up only your share of space. Make only small waves. Respect other peoples' space. As with everything in life, just be considerate.

• **Finally, of course, never, never, never urinate in a pool.** In warm water and experiencing gentle yogic massage of your internal organs, including your intestines, kidneys and bladder, the need to "go" may sneak up on you. Avoid this by emptying your bladder (and bowels, if possible) before you begin WaterYoga. A warm shower may help you "go." You don't want to have to interrupt your WaterYoga practice to use the bathroom.

3. RULES FOR PRACTICING WATERYOGA. These rules are also common sense, subject to your own good judgment.

• **Do too little rather than too much.** Even the mild postures and stretches of WaterYoga may be "too much" at first if you are not used to stretching, or if your body is vulnerable. If you are used to vigorous exercise, or if you like to challenge yourself, you may find the postures and movements so mild that you overdo.

• **Do not stay in the water past your limitation.** You must follow medical advice if you have a problem such as high blood pressure or stroke, or if you are pregnant. Some warm pools advise a general limit of twenty minutes. Some people feel no ill effect from long periods of time in the thermal pool. Others must avoid dizziness, weakness or lethargy by limiting their time. Since being in the water can be dehydrating to the body, a water bottle at poolside is advised. You can become seriously dehydrated without realizing it.

• **Don't compete.** Don't compete with other people. You don't know how long it has taken him or her to develop flexibility. Your body is not like anyone else's body. Don't compare your progress with that of others, sick or well, old or young. If comparison is unavoidable, don't let it grow into competition.

• **Don't set performance goals for yourself.** Experience each WaterYoga practice for itself. Where you are is where you begin. Progress is slow and subtle. Do not expect to make rapid or constant progress. How far and how fast you progress is what YOUR body suggests to you at each practice. Your flexibility or range of motion will vary from practice to practice depending on many circumstances.

You are never finished (never perfectly flexible). Don't be seduced by measurements such as how far, how many, how fast, how often. Your "goal," in the absence of a better term, is only the pleasure of your weightlessness, the grace of your postures and stretches, your body awareness and sense of well-being.

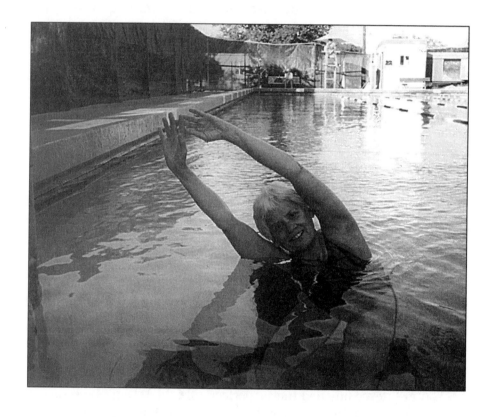

Photograph 6. Jill in Half-Moon. Legs are outlined to help you see the stretch as she stands in shoulder deep water.

PART THREE: GUIDANCE FOR WATERYOGA PRACTICE

If you have found a WaterYoga class, your teacher will explain how the lessons go. If you are on your own, this is an important part for you to read and absorb.

I. GENERAL GUIDANCE FOR PRACTICE TECHNIQUE

• **Start every WaterYoga session quietly.** Spend five or ten minutes acclimating your body to the warmth of the water and to your weight-lessness in it. Stand in shoulder-deep water, observing and enjoying the absence of downward pressure on your back, legs and feet. Feel your shoulders becoming looser. Then support yourself on your noodle: drape your upper arms over it in front of you, parallel to your shoulders, as if you were leaning across the back fence. Hold a second noodle for stability if you like. Bend your legs enough to free your feet from the bottom and find out how completely you can relax. Take three or more deep breaths, staying relaxed. Read the section on breathing to learn how various forms of breathing affect you physically and psychologically.

• **Always go into a basic WaterYoga posture—Mountain or Suspended Zen—before moving on to other postures or stretches.** This way, you conform all of your practice to the principles of good posture and body alignment. Read and re-read the descriptions of Mountain and Suspended Zen in Part Four: WaterYoga Practice. Review these basic postures frequently. Have a professional observe you if you are unsure of your posture and body alignment.

• **Never force any posture or movement past your comfort toler-ance.** Remain in a posture or stretch only as long as you can remain relaxed, as your breathing remains regular, and as it is balanced by the equally pleasant sensation of lengthening and stretching of your muscles and skeleton. Sharp pain, or nerve pain, is an urgent signal to stop because you did something you should not have. A later sec-tion deals at more length with the risks and usefulness of pain in WaterYoga.

There are two observable indicators that you have exceeded your tolerance:

1. Tension in your face, evidenced by grimacing, redness or clenching your jaws. Ease up until your face relaxes.
2. Holding your breath in a posture or stretch. Even under water you should always exhale slowly and steadily.

• **Never bounce against anything to force a stretch.** In the past, bouncing was encouraged when doing floor-based stretching. It was thought to enhance the stretch. Bouncing has now been discredited because of its potential for injury. The present theory is that bouncing sends a message to the muscles to tense up—the exact opposite of the goal of stretching.

Your body is extremely responsive to gentle instruction. It resists violent treatment with equal force. The branch of the autonomic ner-vous system called the sympathetic nervous system evokes the "fight or flight response." It is activated by violent treatment. Substantial bouncing will, therefore, more than likely fill your body with fight-or-flight messages. Out-of-control fight-or-flight messages create a wide range of adverse physiological effects, including inflammation, tension, stiffness and strain. Subtle treatment, on the other hand, will enhance the "rest and repose" response. Don't strive for more.

• **Go slowly into postures and stretches, letting the water do its work.** Feel relaxed and passive, rather than aggressive. Take time to stabilize yourself in each posture. Become aware of your body in it. Direct your mind to the joints and tissues that are involved in each stretch. Breathe into them. This is an esoteric concept for those not experienced in Yoga. Don't worry if it doesn't make sense to you. Your attention to your body will suffice.

• **Breathe throughout a posture or stretch.** Breathing during a posture or stretch is a different concept from "breathing into" a joint or
muscle.

Constant, gentle breathing enhances the relaxation that is the core
of WaterYoga. Do not hold your breath. If you hold your breath, your
muscles and tissues automatically tend to contract and stiffen, which
interferes with the deepening of the posture.

Breathe quietly. Tension, both physical and emotional, are closely
related to breathing patterns. Quick, high, shallow breathing indicates
tension, while slow, deep, steady breathing indicates serenity and
calm alertness. Your brain reads audible breathing as a stress (fight-
or-flight) signal and tells your muscles to mobilize (become tense) for
defense.

The rib cage is often an area of tension. This tension is directly
related to restrictions in breathing. As the muscles around the rib cage
release, the rib cage becomes freer, and breathing improves naturally.

The diaphragm is the partition between the chest and the
abdomen. When it is restricted by the abdominal muscles, it cannot
move down into the abdomen on inhalation. For deep breathing, the
abdomen should visibly rise and fall.

This rule applies as well if your head is under water: let your lungs
slowly and continuously exhale. The more you can relax the longer you
will be able to hold the stretch before coming up for breath.

• **Try to hold each posture or stretch for at least 30 seconds.** It
can take healthy, relaxed muscles that long to "let go." Letting go happens when the muscle itself seems to come to understand what is
wanted of it. Experienced yoga practitioners often actually feel the
moment when their muscles relax. Do not worry if you don't feel it. Be
patient and conscientious, but never expect anything to happen. You
can't make it happen. Trying to make it happen leads to stress—the
very opposite of relaxation. When you feel the letting-go you may deep-
en the posture or stretch. Or, you may be content and move on to the
next posture or stretch.

- **Don't hurry!** Take time to absorb the last stretch before introducing the next one. Heed the ancient Chinese saying: "Wait for three breaths before going to the next thing."

- **Allow time for your body to heal.** Modify your postures if you are recovering from the acute phase of any physical problem, or from a set-back.

- **Be creative.** As you educate yourself about your own body and its needs and limitations, you will undoubtedly personalize your WaterYoga practice. Adapt what you see others doing to your own needs. Invent a new posture. Every practitioner is both teacher and student.

- **Finish positively.** Take a few minutes to let your body feel the joy of the WaterYoga experience before you take your new awareness out of the water and into life.

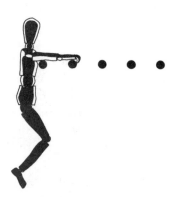

II. THE ROLE OF PAIN

As you practice WaterYoga, as in all the activities of your life, you must learn to distinguish various kinds of pain. Pain is always a messenger. You must learn to heed the message. The message of pain is so important that it deserves its own section. I have synthesized this section from the insights of three people whose work I credit here. Mary Pullig Schatz, M.D., discusses the various kinds of pain more fully in her book, BACK CARE BASICS, A DOCTOR'S GENTLE YOGA PROGRAM FOR BACK AND NECK PAIN RELIEF.

• **Bad pain.** Any movement that creates numbness, twinges or sharp burning pain signals a harmful movement. Stop. Don't try to "work through" bad pain. The harsh days of "no pain, no gain" are gone.

Judith Stransky writes in ALEXANDER TECHNIQUE, THE JOY IN THE LIFE OF YOUR BODY, that pain is a "telephone" call from the body, an SOS, a call for help. And taking an aspirin or some other pain killer is like taking the telephone off the hook. As Ms. Stransky says, we should listen to the message that bad pain sends, loud and clear: misuse of the body.

There are other clues that you are risking misuse. Back off if your jaws clench or your face distorts, or your normal breathing is interrupted.

• **Useful pain.** Trigger point pain can be useful. It is also a sharp "twinging" pain. Stop immediately if you experience this kind of pain. Though bad, it may identify the "trigger point" for referred pain. Because the trigger point is not necessarily the same place where you feel the pain, locating it can be very helpful in assessing a physical problem.

• **Good pain.** In contrast to the twinges and burning of bad pain, the sensation of muscle stretch is a good one, a subtle combination of pleasure and discomfort, perhaps a good "hurt," but not truly a pain. You can tell you are feeling the "good pain" of stretch if you are doing the posture or stretch without facial distortion and without interrupting your normal breathing. Gloria Carpeneto, my massage therapist, tells me that some people tell her, "Oh, this hurts good."

• **Post-practice pain.** I prefer to call this good pain "soreness" or "stiffness." After a WaterYoga practice you may have some soreness and stiffness. If you have worked hard, or tried new stretches, this is normal and expected. It is the same kind of stiffness you experience after any strenuous exercise. If it is mild and abates in a day, it is probably good. If it lasts for more than a day or two, you have done too much. Soften up your practice. Many experts prefer a cycle of alternate days of rest and activity to let the body recover. And read up on lactate buildup and anti-oxidants.

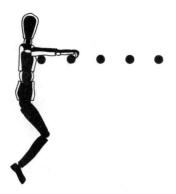

PART FOUR: WATERYOGA PRACTICE

The postures and stretches of WaterYoga are divided into sections that are determined by the depth of the water in which you practice WaterYoga. Section II–Plus is not, strictly speaking, WaterYoga, but its gentle motions follow naturally from WaterYoga stretches. The fifth section is the shower, where you can benefit from warm water, if not from weightlessness. Part Five is specially devoted to care of the back while it is in spasm. It describes the postures and stretches that I used to lull my back out of spasm.

I. Standing on the Bottom in Chest-Deep Water
I–Plus. Standing on the Bottom at a Wall in Chest-Deep Water

II. Suspended on Noodles in at Least Chest-Deep Water
II–Plus. Gentle Movements From WaterYoga Stretches

III. In Shallow Water

IV. In Any Depth of Water

V. In the Shower

See PART FIVE for Back Spasm: Special Practice

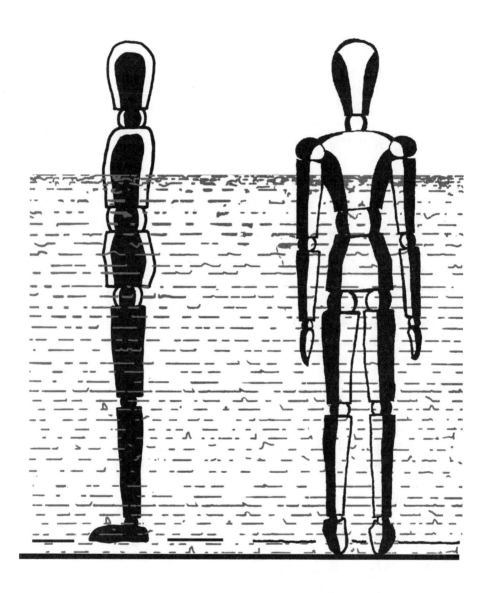

Illustration 7. Mountain Pose, side and front views. This is the starting posture for stretches standing in chest deep water. Look back at Illustration 2 on page 21 to visualize how your body masses and your bones conform to this posture.

SECTION I. STANDING IN CHEST-DEEP WATER

MOUNTAIN POSE: THE STARTING POINT

Your body has three main bulky parts: head, thorax and pelvis. Thorax and pelvis together are the trunk, or torso, but back flexibility allows them to move somewhat independently. In good posture, these three parts are properly aligned, so that their muscles do not have to work hard to keep them from succumbing to the pull of gravity.

In humans, the axis of gravity passes down the middle of the spinal curves. The lumbar spine takes up most of the back half of the trunk. The thoracic spine also extends deeply toward the center. Contrary to what most of us think, the spine really is near the middle of the body mass. It does not lie on the surface of the back. In good posture, the gravity axis passes down the middle of the head, thorax and pelvis, down the legs and through both ends of the arches of the feet to the floor.

In recent years, a Yoga Master named B.K.S. Iyengar has greatly influenced the practice of Hatha Yoga. He observed that good posture is directly related to good health. Therefore, all Iyengar Yoga postures aim to align the head, neck, shoulders, spine, hips, knees and feet in good posture.

Because all body parts are interrelated, improper alignment of one adversely affects all the others. For instance, a forward-thrust head becomes the counterweight for abnormal curve in the lower spine, with resultant strain on both muscular and skeletal systems.

A strained high-shouldered posture, in which chest and shoulder muscles pull (contract) toward the neck, raises the scapulae along with the shoulders. The powerful neck muscles in the back tend to contract, compressing the cervical vertebrae. I know people whose necks have seemed to disappear.

If the chest is carried too far forward and too high, increased lordosis (Greek: bending backward) may result. When chest muscles are too tense, they compress the spine. The crowded vertebrae have nowhere to go but out, making a hump at the back of the neck or a rounded back. Conversely, when the upper spine is overly curved, hunched, or rounded, the chest slumps. When the lumbar curve is exaggerated in swayback, there is often a compensating exaggerated curve elsewhere: neck, thoracic spine, or even hyperextension in the knees. Whenever any spinal curve is exaggerated, the height of the torso is decreased.

Poor posture also affects the internal organs. When the length of the thoracic spine decreases, it diminishes the available space in the chest cavity for the heart and lungs. When the heart and lungs are

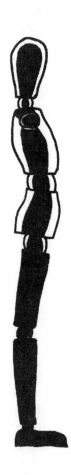

forced to displace themselves downward toward the stomach and abdomen, the abdominal cavity becomes overcrowded. The damage is reciprocal because the overcrowding puts additional strain on the abdominal muscles, which must hold the abdominal organs that lie above the pelvic bowl. It is not surprising that a protruding abdomen often accompanies a slumped upper body.

Whenever the pelvis, thorax or head is unbalanced on the axis of gravity, its bony weight puts unnatural strain on the muscles of the back and abdomen. Lack of support from weakened abdominal muscles puts additional strain on the spine, exacerbating the postural problem.

WaterYoga seeks to reeducate the body to align posture as much as possible along its center of gravity. You can practice in your morning shower when you can't get to a warm water facility. I have added my voice to three others that address the same theory of posture.

Illustration 8. Incorrect Mountain Pose. This view shows swayback but without compensating forward thrust of the head. It also shows hyperextended knees, which may throw the pelvis forward to compensate for changing the gravitational axis.

- **Mountain Pose**. Mountain is the basic pose for most yoga practice. It is called "Mountain" because it represents stability and solidity and yet reaches for the sky.

1. Stand in chest-deep water, with your feet about eighteen inches apart, and balance your body equally on both feet. Stabilize yourself by resting your hands on a noodle in front of you, if it makes you more comfortable. Breathe normally.
2. Curve your spine naturally. Do not accentuate the curve in your lower back, or tuck your buttocks under you to flatten your back.
3. Bring your shoulders down and apart, hanging loose and relaxed. At the same time raise your upper sternum, being careful not to poke your lower ribs out in front. Drop your scapulae down your back. Keep them wide. Be sure they do not strain toward your spine or up toward your ears.
4. Elongate your spine, lowering your sacrum. At the same time, sense your hip bones lifting up, away from your thigh bones, your waist from your hips, your rib cage from your waist, each vertebra separating from its lower neighbor. Be aware of how easy this is to do in the water. Hold your thorax and pelvis well together, using psoas and other deep inner abdominal muscles as well as the muscles of your abdominal wall. Feel your trunk as one piece.
5. Lengthen your neck, vertebra by vertebra. Bring your chin toward the back of your head without hardening your throat. Keep your head level and well up from your shoulders. Keep your neck straight. The yogi believe this allows the Ch'i to flow up into your brain.
6. Feel how elongating your spine and lifting your sternum maximize the space that holds your internal organs.
7. Activate your diaphragm and abdominal muscles. Be aware of your lungs filling the additional space as you breathe. But do not flare out your lower ribs. Keep your torso narrow and tall. Feel your diaphragm lift and make more room for your intestines. Feel your abdominal muscles holding your intestines in your pelvic bowl and helping the muscles of your back support your spine.
8. Feel your feet resting on the bottom while your head rises upward, as if you have grown two inches taller.
9. Be sure that you do not hyperextend your knees, which is to lock them at a slight angle toward your back.
10. Maintain this posture, breathing quietly for at least a minute. This will imprint it as you go into other postures and stretches.

• **The Dinosaur of Mabel E. Todd**. Mabel E. Todd published a book
called THE THINKING BODY in 1937, setting out a theory of posture
based on the physics of human anatomy. Ms. Todd says: ***"Think
down the back and up the front."*** Thinking "up the front" of the
body activates the supporting abdominal muscles and sets the posture
of the thorax and pelvis in balance to support the organs that are suspended from the spine. Thinking "down the back" means to let the
spine drag, extended, as Ms. Todd said, like a dinosaur's tail. In this
posture the muscles and ligaments of the spine best maintain the natural curves of the spine.

The dinosaur's axis passes through his pelvis. His whole upper
body is counterbalanced by his enormous heavy tail.

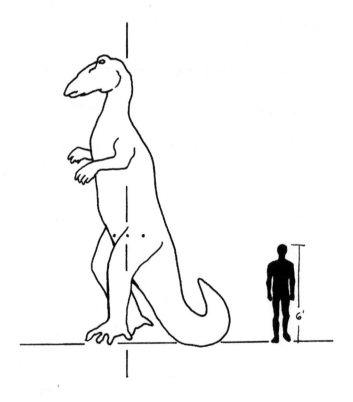

Illustration 9. Dinosaur. This is a friendly vegetarian dinosaur, who
reaches high up into the trees to feed on leaves. Notice how immense
his tail must be to balance his heavy abdomen and thighs, and how
his tail peters out at the end to match his small forelegs and head.
His axis of gravity, too, seems balanced over his pelvis.

• **Alexander Technique.** The Alexander Technique concentrates on the head and neck in educating the body to stand and move in good posture. It is a conscious learning process, built on giving one's self instructions, rather than doing anything physical. The instructions are the words that Matthias Alexander used, to be said like a mantra:

LET THE NECK BE FREE,

TO LET THE HEAD GO FORWARD AND UP,

TO LET THE BACK LENGTHEN AND WIDEN.

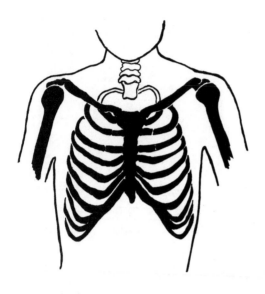

view a.

Illustration 10. Front views of ribs, sternum, clavicles and arms. The top of the sternum is the only bony connection of the shoulder/arm system to the rest of the skeleton. Notice that the clavicles are essentially horizontal in view b. So is the top rib.

In view a, the shoulders have been raised and hunched, and the top rib canted toward the front. All of this has the effect of shortening the appearance of the neck.

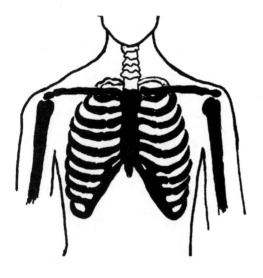

view b.

• **Lampshade, the Image That Helps Me Understand Posture.** I look at my clavicles as the latch-key to good posture. Did the Romans know this when they called the collar bone the "clavicle," or "small key?" Only the clavicles connect the shoulder girdle to the rest of the skeleton. All the rest of the shoulder girdle, from which hang our very useful and active arms, float free of it. In good posture the clavicles should be nearly horizontal.

The lampshade image of your upper body and shoulders may seem as unlikely as Ms. Todd's dinosaur until I describe a lamp in my living room. It has a rectangular shade, which is attached by wire cross pieces, or struts, to a circle of metal that is attached to a central post. Two lights are cantilevered (side-loaded, as Ms. Mabel Todd would say) on the central post. The broad lamp-base is like a pelvis. The finial at the top is like a slender, erect neck rising from the post. It is an almost perfect image of the shoulder girdle and torso.

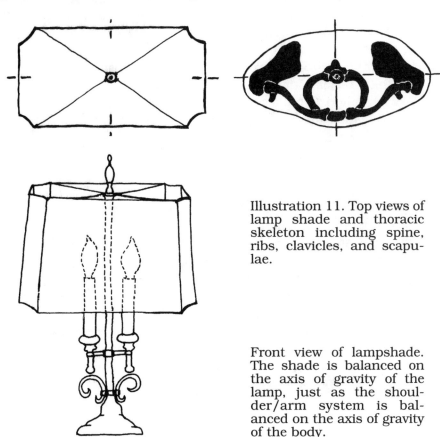

Illustration 11. Top views of lamp shade and thoracic skeleton including spine, ribs, clavicles, and scapulae.

Front view of lampshade. The shade is balanced on the axis of gravity of the lamp, just as the shoulder/arm system is balanced on the axis of gravity of the body.

This is the image I see: the axis of gravity runs up the post, like a spine; the shade floats free from the light bulbs like a shoulder girdle; it is connected to the lamp itself only by struts like clavicles; and most importantly to both esthetics and function, the struts are horizontal, just as the clavicles should be.

• Lampshade Pose

1. Stand in Mountain. Trace the length of your clavicles with your fingers to see how nearly horizontally they stretch from your sternum to the tips of your shoulders. If you have access to a mirror, you can see them beneath the skin.
2. Think of your upper body as a lamp and your shoulder girdle as its shade. The small metal circle is your top ribs, connected at the back to your spine and at the front to the top of your sternum. Lift the top of your sternum to make the circle horizontal. If the circle tips away from the horizontal, the lampshade will go awry, caving in your chest and rounding your back, or allowing an arm to press against your rib cage. Think about the finial rising up as you raise your neck and head.
3. Think of the horizontal struts that hold the lampshade as the clavicles that anchor your shoulder bones to your sternum. Drop your clavicles to horizontal, feeling your shoulders widen.
4. Raise the outer tips of your shoulders up as far as you can. Notice that their upward angle narrows your shoulders and crowds your neck. Notice how this changes the relation between your chin and your shoulder joints.
5. Drop your shoulders back down and feel them relax, free from your chest and ribs, like the lampshade on its metal struts, the clavicles that connect your shoulders to the rest of your skeleton.
6. Raise your shoulders again. Think how bad the lampshade would look if the struts were bent up so much that they hid the beautiful finial.
7. Drop your shoulders again, being aware of how this frees your neck to be longer.
8. Center the lampshade over the post; that is, balance your shoulder girdle on your axis of gravity, side to side and front to back. Feel how your arms hang free, not pressing on your rib cage.
9. Breathe way down into your abdomen. Your shoulders don't have to help you breathe.

STRETCHES FROM MOUNTAIN POSE

Flexibility requires long elastic muscles. Tight muscles and inelastic connective tissues put unnatural pressure on the bones. Anger, tension, pain, injury, over-use, strain, surgery, and the inevitable process of aging can all cause the muscles to tighten. Bones that are too closely bound together together eventually grind against each other, wearing away important joint cartilage. This leads to abrasion and pain. Pain signals the muscles to constrict even further. The damaging effect is cyclical. Loosening the muscles and connective tissues can stop the cycle.

Because all of the parts of the body are related, tight muscles in one part put strain on the rest. Here are two examples.

If your hips are immobile, you strain your vertebrae because you must bend your back to lean forward. Tight hips are often not an obvious problem, like a "bad back," but can be the hidden source of a back problem. I think this was part of my own experience. Loosening the hips so they act as a hinge for bending forward decreases the strain on the back.

If the chest muscles are too tight, the shoulders are drawn forward, rounding the upper back and pitching the neck forward as well. Loosening the chest can free the back to straighten.

The following stretches are a quiet and efficient way of increasing flexibility.

BACK STRETCHES FROM MOUNTAIN POSE

Establish yourself in Mountain for a few minutes. Focus your body and mind on proper posture before you practice your standing WaterYoga stretches.

- **Half-Moon.**
1. Raise both arms above your head, stretching your body as tall as possible.
2. Slowly curve the whole length of your body to the right, as if you were the new moon. Try to keep the curve constant. Hold. Feel the stretch on your left side from shoulder to thigh and the corresponding contraction on the right side.
3. Intensify if you feel comfortable. Return to Mountain.
4. Repeat, curving to the left.

Illustration 12. Half Moon

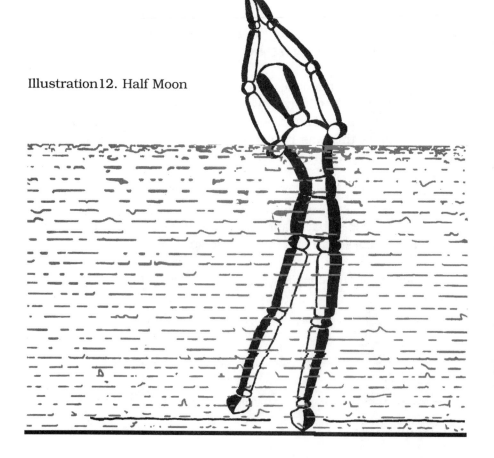

• **Arch/Slump.** Whenever you do any movement or exercise in which you bend backwards, complement the backward stretch by a forward stretch.

1. Support your lower back by placing the palms of your hands on your back, just below the waist, little fingers together and fingers spread. Your thumbs should ride on the tops of your hips. Instruct your back to lengthen as you bend backwards.

2. Keeping your shoulders low, arch your back and raise your sternum and your chin.

3. Hold, breathing normally. Feel your back muscles at work.

4. Return to Mountain and shift your hands so that your thumbs are at the back, on the tops of your hips, and your fingers are at the sides of your abdomen.

5. Keeping your shoulders low and wide and your spine long, round each vertebra forward, starting at the top of your neck and working downward. If your face goes under water, your feet will float up. That is all right, but you may prefer to limit the forward bend to keep your face out of the water.

6. Return to Mountain.

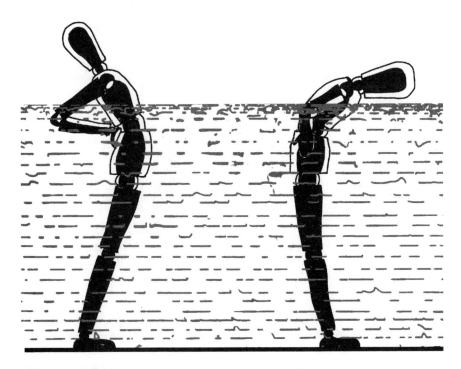

Illustration 13. Arch/Slump

• **Twist, Mountain.** Your spine has no major joint that allows it to twist easily, the way the elbows, wrists, and shoulders do. In addition, your back muscles are not very elastic, which is why they hurt if you try to stretch them too much. In water, however, there is minimal risk of strain during the Twist. You may even find greater flexibility in your back because the vertebrae are not compressed by your body's weight on them. Nevertheless, do not push the Twist past your comfort zone.

1. Slowly rotate your shoulders to the right, allowing your chest to follow. Stabilize with a noodle if you like.
2. Allow your lower trunk and hips to follow your chest to the right.
3. Turn your head to the right, keeping it level and centered. Be sure to follow the suggestions in the Neck Stretches section.
4. Hold and return to Mountain.
5. Repeat to the left.

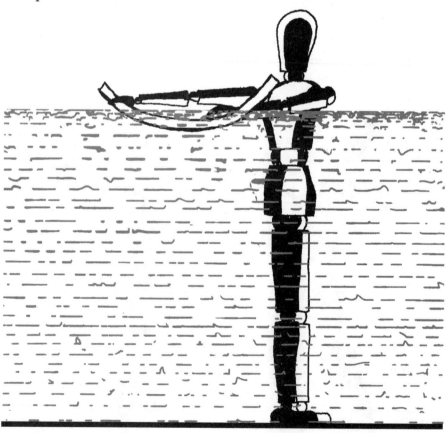

Illustration 14. Twist, Mountain. Notice that head turns to left, feet turn to right.

NECK STRETCHES FROM MOUNTAIN POSE

The head can weigh more than fifteen pounds. Simplified for purposes of this discussion, it has two bones, the skull and the lower jaw.

Occipital condyles (nubs under the base of the skull) allow the skull to rock backward and forward on corresponding projections of the Atlas, which is the top, or first, cervical (neck) vertebra. The Atlas is named for Atlas, a powerful giant, son of Titan, of Greek mythology. Old maps show Atlas kneeling, carrying the world on his shoulders. That is why old maps, then books of maps were called "atlases." The Atlas mountains in North Africa, the Atlantic ocean, and the lost continent of Atlantis are all named for him.

The world bears very heavily on Atlas's shoulders as he rocks his head forward to accept the load. Just think of all that history resting on the base of your own skull!

Rocking your skull on your atlas creates the motion of nodding "yes" that is important to the Alexander Technique. It occurs at the center of the base of the skull, at a level just below the ear lobes, not at the back of your neck. It is important to understand this rocking movement, and distinguish it from a hinge movement, like the hip.

The position and shape of the condyles limit the range of rocking motion by the skull on the atlas and also prevent side-bending and rotation at that level of the neck.

Rotation occurs largely at the joint of the atlas and second cervical vertebra, which is called the axis. In rotation, the atlas pivots on the axis to create the "no" motion. Rotation is limited to about 90 degrees to each side. This means that you cannot comfortably turn your head past the line of your shoulders.

Side-bending occurs for the most part at the joints of the cervical vertebrae below the axis.

Because of this division of labor among the cervical vertebrae, many experts feel that neck circles (circumduction) are not a good exercise. I do not include them here.

In good posture, the side-to-side center of the head sits directly over the center of the atlas-axis joint. If not centered, it would over-work the supporting neck and back muscles.

From front to back, however, more of the weight of the head sits in front of the cervical spine than in back. This weight is counterbalanced by powerful muscles in the back of the neck. A too-forward jutting head overworks those muscles. The strain of this posture can intensi-fy rounded shoulders. It can also cause the cervical and thoracic ver-tebrae to slide forward on their lower neighbors, creating a harmful shearing force.

Your neck muscles link your skull to your shoulder bones and spine. Your jaw muscles affect your temples and the musculature of the spine. This means that head pain can develop from tension in the back and vice versa.

Although neck stretches are best done in Mountain, you may do them anywhere you can comfortably submerge the muscles in your neck. And you can do them in the shower.

Always do neck stretches very gently and precisely so as not to cre-ate any pain. Remember that all neck stretches must be very gently. AS IN ALL WATERYOGA, DO NOT BOUNCE. Be especially cautious if you have any orthopedic or neural problems in your neck.

Start from Mountain. Keep your clavicles and shoulders in good posture.

- **Atlas Rocking.**
1. Balance your head over the spinal axis.
2. Make a small nodding "yes" motion for a few moments.
3. Put a finger on each side of your neck just below your ears to locate the atlas as you continue to nod. Feel with your fingers which muscles are involved in rocking.
4. Gently "float" your head up from this level, keeping your forehead and chin in a single vertical plane.
5. Feel your head—your mental "world"—rock easily, cradled on the broad base of the atlas. Feel the freedom in your neck muscles.

- **Crane.** This is an intensification of Atlas Rocking.
6. Slide your chin forward on your atlas. Hold.
7. Drop your chin down to your sternum. Hold
8. Draw your neck back softly, but maintaining the position of your vertebrae that you have established. Hold.
9. Raise your chin to the position of step 4 and 5.

- **Axis Turning.**
1. Allow your head to float up and away from your shoulders.
2. Keeping your head high and level, your neck long, your chin tucked in, and your throat relaxed, slowly turn your head to the right. Feel with your fingers which muscles are involved in turning. Hold
3. Return to Mountain, and repeat on the left.

- **Neck Bending.**
1. Allow your head to float up and away from your shoulders.
2. Keeping your head high, your neck long, your chin tucked in and your throat relaxed, lower your forehead slowly toward your left shoulder. Feel the pull in the muscles on the right side of your neck. Feel them with your fingers. If your have a mirror you may see them. Visualize which vertebrae are moving and how. Hold.
3. Return to vertical. Repeat on the right.
4. As an intensification of this stretch, rotate your chin slowly back and down toward your shoulder (DO NOT raise your shoulder toward your chin.) Feel the lengthening of the powerful back-of-the-neck muscles that support your head.

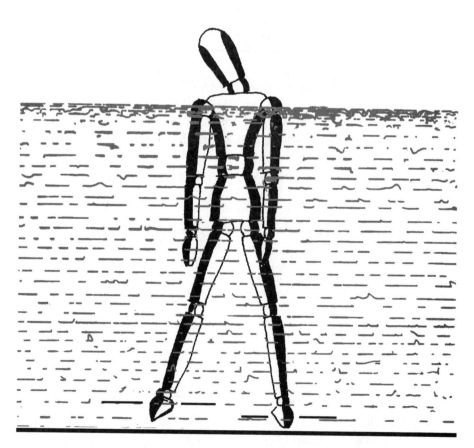

Illustration 15. Neck Bending

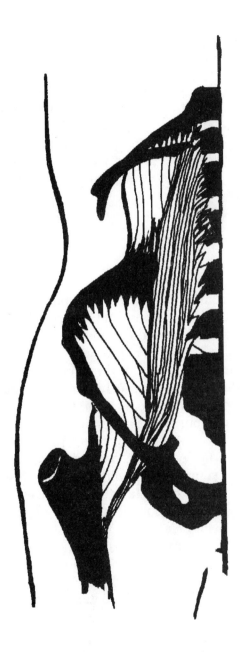

Illustration 16. Psoas and iliopsoas muscles, front view of right side. Together they form a major muscle system in the interior of the abdomen, connecting the lower ribs and pelvis to the thigh.

HIP OPENERS FROM MOUNTAIN POSE

Your pelvis is the bony part of the bowl that contains your abdominal organs. Pelvis means "bowl" in Latin. It is composed of the sacrum, coccyx, ilia, and pubic bone. The frontal abdominal muscles complete the bowl. The tilt of the pelvis is determined by the muscles of the hips and the abdomen (flexors, hamstrings and under-regarded iliopsoas, which runs in front of the spine and extends all the way from the thigh to the diaphragm). Proper posture and movement require flexibility in the hip joints and strength in the abdominal muscles.

• **Pelvis Rock.** This stretch will make you aware of the relation between your pelvis and your spinal curve.
1. Spread your feet comfortably to stabilize your balance.
2. Gently rub your lower back (waist and below) with the backs of both hands, diagonally down toward the middle.
3. Put the fingers of both hands across your lower back, thumbs on your hips, at the crest, or top of the bone, and slowly shift your pelvis backward. Imagine your pelvic bowl tipping toward your back, sloshing out Champagne, if you prefer not to imagine it sloshing out viscera. Feel your back flatten. To counterbalance this, your coccyx, or "tail-bone," will shift forward. (Your "sit-bones" may or may not move. (Sit-bones are the two knobs that you can feel with your hands under your buttocks when you sit. This is an accurate name, related to the German "sitz." Anatomically they are called ischial tuberosities.) Feel your buttocks ("glutes") and abdominal muscles tighten. Hold. Relax.
4. Slowly shift your pelvis forward, sloshing the Champagne or viscera out the front of the bowl. Notice that this increases the curve (lordosis) of your lower back. Hold. Feel your lower back muscles tighten. Relax. Be aware of the range of motion in your pelvis.

• **Tree.** Hold a noodle at arm's length to stabilize your body if it helps.
1. Place your right foot against the inside of your left thigh, as high up as possible.
2. Keeping your pelvis stable, swing your knee to the right. Hold.
3. Release and repeat with your left leg.

Illustration 17. Tree

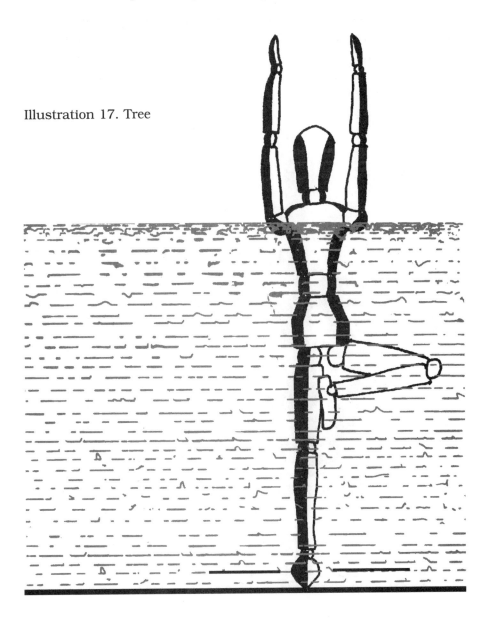

• **Stork.** This stretch will also strengthen your arms. Hold a noodle at arm's length to stabilize your body.

1. Pick up the top of your right foot in your right hand.
2. Keeping your pelvis stable, and your knees in the same sideways plane, lift your right foot toward your right buttock. Hold.
3. Release and repeat with your left leg.

Illustration 18. Stork

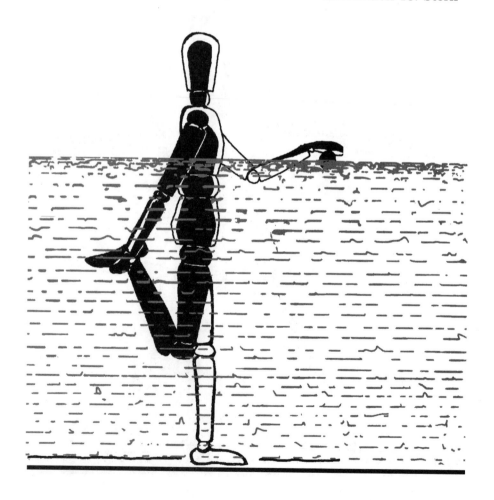

- **Five Pointed Star.** In this basic stretch, you imagine yourself pressed between two sheets of glass.
1. Stretch both arms straight out to the sides, horizontal and activated. Feel your shoulders as wide as possible, your fingertips pulled to the walls (horizon) on either side of you. Feel your shoulders down, your clavicles horizontal.
2. Spread your legs to the sides as far as possible. Feel them pulled to the floor on either side of you, straight and activated, your kneecaps raised. Feel your head floating upward toward the sky (ceiling) and your coccyx dragging downward.
3. Rotate your thighs, calves and feet outward, maintaining the breadth of spread apart. Hold.
4. Return to Mountain.

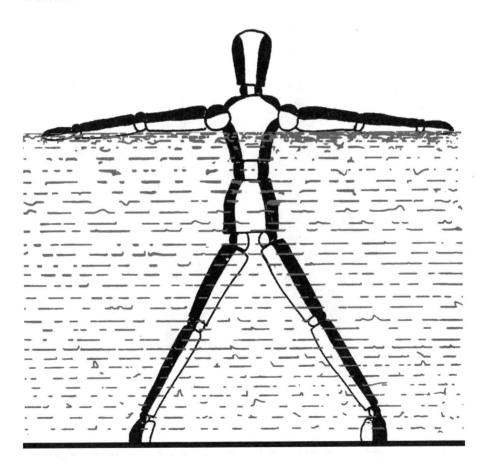

Illustration 19. Five Pointed Star.

SHOULDER STRETCHES FROM MOUNTAIN POSE

Remember to keep your clavicles horizontal and your shoulders relaxed, down and wide (except in Shrug).

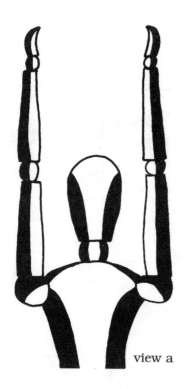 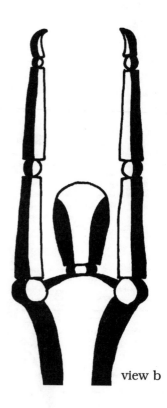

view a   view b

Illustration 20. Movement of the shoulders in raising the arms. View a shows correct movement, and view b shows incorrect movement for yoga. Even though the figure can reach a little higher, the neck and shoulder muscles are constricted. Notice how much longer the neck is and how much more space there is between the head and shoulders in view a.

- **Prayer.**
1. Raise both arms straight out to the sides at shoulder height.
2. Bend your elbows to raise your forearms to the vertical.
3. Bring your forearms together vertically in front of your chest. Hold.
4. Return to Mountain.
5. As an intensification of this stretch, intertwine your forearms, lacing your fingers together.

- **Prayer Circles.** Prayer circles are a continuation of Prayer.
6. Inhaling, slowly raise both arms slowly up and out. Feel your upper chest rise.
7. Exhaling, rotate your hands downward and toward the back, keeping your arms straight. Feel your scapulae (shoulder blades) drop down your back.
8. Squeeze your scapulae together.
9. Repeat 1 through 8 slowly, matching your movements to your breathing pattern.

Illustration 21. Prayer

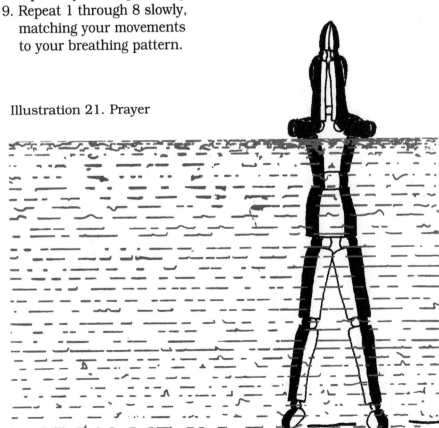

- **Shrug.** Review illustration 20 because in Shrug you move through the shoulder postions in view a and view b.
1. Lift both shoulders toward your ears. Hold.
2. Move both shoulders forward as far as possible. Hold.
3. Drop both shoulders back to Mountain.
4. Repeat as is comfortable.

- **Shoulder Hinge.**
1. Extend your right arm straight out in front of you, palm inward.
2. Slowly bring your right elbow as far as possible toward your left shoulder. Support it with your left arm and apply only as much pressure as is comfortable. Hold.
3. Return to Mountain.
4. Repeat with left arm.

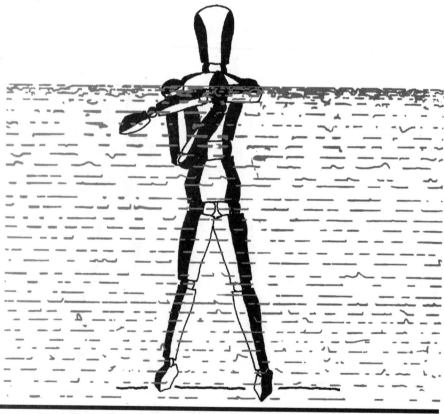

Illustration 22. Shoulder Hinge

• **Street Light.** In this stretch your profile *might* look like a street light. (This stretch could do with a better title. Ideas are welcome.)
1. With arms straight, lace your fingers together behind your back.
2. Turn your palms out and down.
3. Keeping your arms straight, raise your hands up behind you. Hold.
4. Return to Mountain.

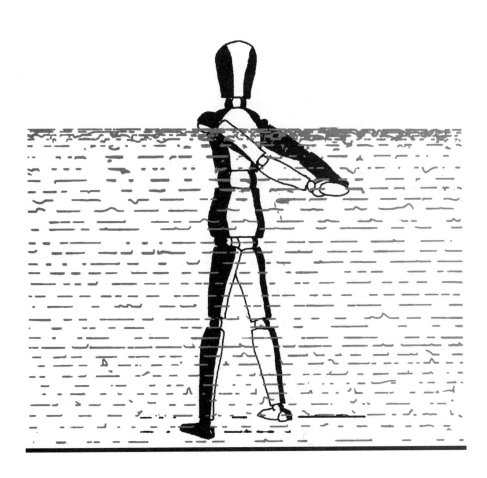

Illustration 23. Street Light

• **Snake Charmer.** You will probably need a noodle to connect your hands in order to complete this stretch.

1. Raise your right arm straight out in front of you, at shoulder height (holding the noodle, palm facing up).
2. Lift your right hand forward, over your head, and drop it behind you so that your hand, holding the noodle, dangles down the middle of your back.

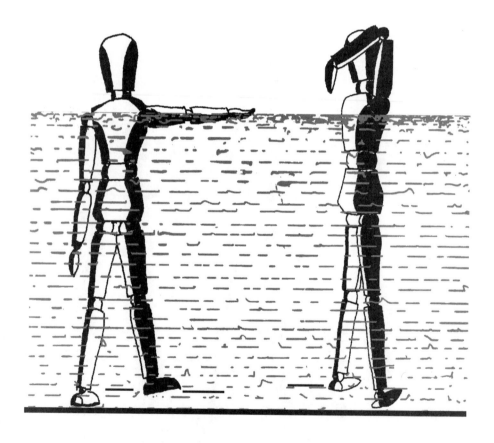

Illustration 24. Snake Charmer. A series of four drawings guides you into this stretch.

- **Snake Charmer, continued.**
3. Raise your left hand, shoulder height, straight out to the side.
4. Rotate your left upper arm forward in the shoulder socket, so that your palm faces backward.
5. Let your left lower arm drop to vertical.
6. Move your left hand to the middle of your back.
7. Grasp the noodle, and work your hands as close together as possible. Only very limber people can grasp one hand with the other without using the noodle. Hold.
8. Return to Mountain.

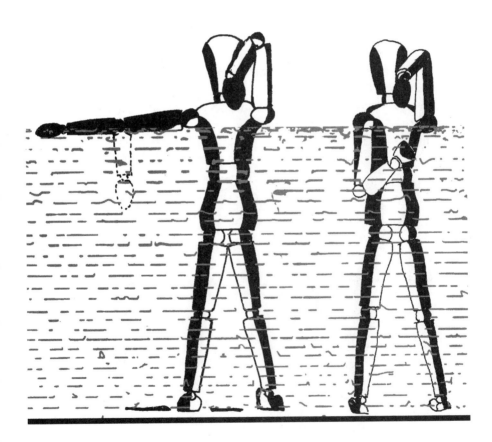

- **Quadrilateral.** This stretch addresses the limited range of shoulder motion that stops you from raising your arms straight above your head. Submerge your shoulders long enough to warm them.
1. Slide your scapulae down your back, and lift your upper sternum and clavicles. Keep your shoulders relaxed and down and wide. Do not hunch them by your ears.
2. Raise both arms straight out to your sides.
3. Turn your palms up. Then turn them down. Sense your shoulder joints opening.
4. Grasp the ends of a noodle in your hands. You may have to bend your arms a little.
5. Slowly lift your hands above your head.
6. Walk your hands as close together on the noodle as you are able. Your arms, the noodle and your shoulders form a quadrilateral. Hold.
7. If you feel a letting go, inch your hands closer together on the noodle. Hold.
8. Release the noodle from one hand and return your arms to horizontal.
9. Return to Mountain.

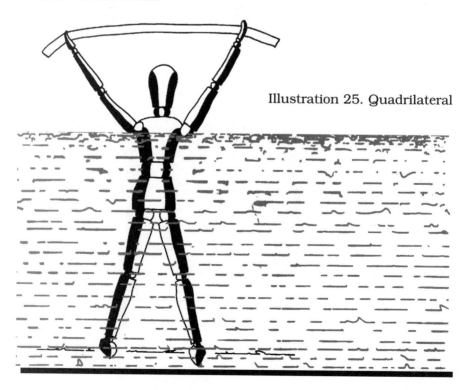

Illustration 25. Quadrilateral

LEG STRETCHES FROM MOUNTAIN POSE

The following stretches address tightness in the hip joints. Hip suppleness is important in reducing the strain on your back when you bend forward.

• **Achilles Stretch A**. Water must be no more than chest deep, so you can keep your nose and mouth above water as you complete this stretch.
1. Keeping your torso erect, bend your knees and ankles as far as you comfortably can. Feel the stretch in your Achilles tendons.
2. Hold and return to Mountain.

Illustration 26. Achilles Stretch A

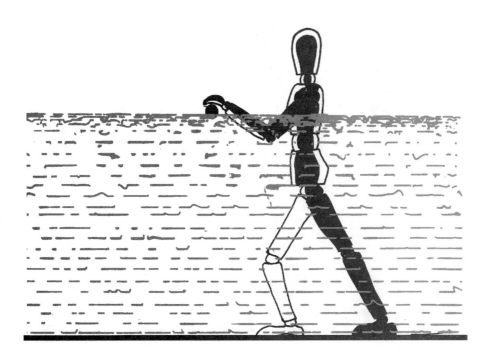

- **Passive Straight Leg Raise.** You will need a noodle.
1. Loop the noodle under your right ankle, holding both ends with your hands.
2. Holding your pelvis level, let the buoyancy of the noodle lift your straight right leg in front of you. For more lift, use two noodles. Hold.
3. Alternate pointing your toes and flexing your ankles. See ankle stretches.
4. Return to Mountain and repeat with your left leg.

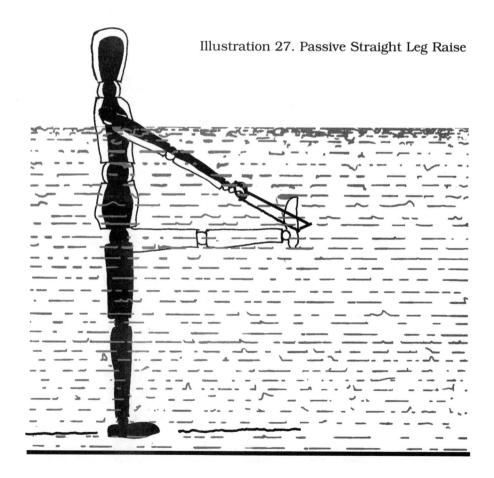

Illustration 27. Passive Straight Leg Raise

- **Active Straight Leg Raise.** This stretch will also tone the muscles in your leg.
1. Holding your pelvis level,, lift your straight right leg in front of you. Hold.
2. Alternate pointing your toes and flexing your ankles. See ankle stretches.
3. Return to Mountain and repeat with your left leg.

- **Passive Bent Leg Raise.** You will need a noodle.
1. Loop the noodle under your right thigh, holding both ends with your hands.
2. Holding your pelvis level, let the buoyancy of the noodle lift your thigh in front of you. For more lift, use two noodles. Hold.
3. Alternate pointing your toes and flexing your ankles. And see ankle stretches.
4. Return to Mountain and repeat with your left leg.

Illustration 28. Passive Bent Leg Raise

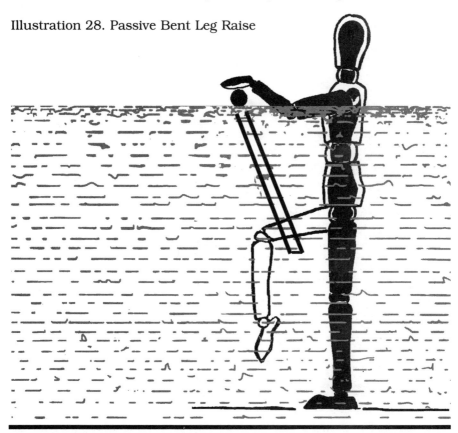

- **Active Bent Leg Raise.** This stretch will also tone the muscles in your thigh.
1. Holding your pelvis level, lift your thigh in front of you, keeping your lower leg parallel to your body. Hold.
2. Alternate pointing your toes and flexing your ankles. See ankle stretches.
3. Return to Mountain and repeat with your left leg.

- **Side Leg Raise.** This is a continuation of all the leg raises.
1. Swing the leg as far to your side as you can, without bending or twisting your back or taking your pelvis out of its level position.

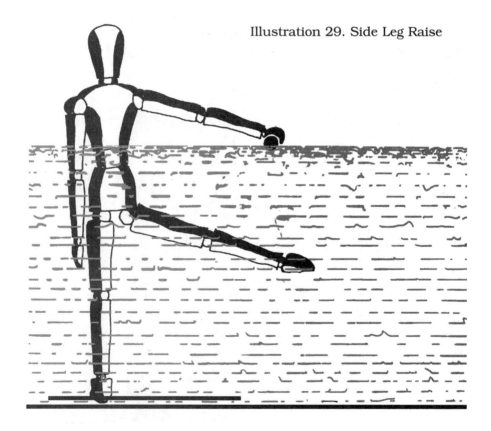

Illustration 29. Side Leg Raise

DIARY OF WATERYOGA PRACTICE

The following two pages are a diary for you to use in keeping track of your WaterYoga practice. You may photocopy these pages as often as you like. (Each two pages make one 8 1/2 by 11 inch page.) If you are working with a health care provider or teacher, that person may want to use this Diary to review your practice with you.

Check off each posture and stretch that you choose to do as part of your WaterYoga practice and note the dates. Make your beginning assessment as complete has possible, because it is so easy to forget details as you progress in your practice. In addition to height and weight, etc., say as much as you can about your flexibility in each of your joints, how long you hold the postures and stretches, any pain or stiffness, and whether one side is different from the other. Describe your posture and muscle tone. You might even have someone take pictures. Describe your balance and breathing. Note the duration of the practice period. Record any other detail of your health that is important to you, like digestion or sleep, for instance.

You will probably need more paper as you make ongoing comments about each posture or stretch, and general observations.

If you are like me, you will also write all over the margins everywhere in this book, expressing agreement or disagreement with it.

DIARY OF WATERYOGA PRACTICE
FIRST LIST: CHEST-DEEP WATER

PRACTICE DATE																	
Mountain																	
Dinosaur																	
Alexander Technique																	
Lampshade																	
Half Moon																	
Arch/Slump																	
Twist, Mountain																	
Atlas Rocking																	
Crane																	
Axis Turning																	
Neck Bending																	
Pelvis Rock																	
Tree																	
Stork																	
Five Pointed Star																	
Prayer																	
Prayer Circles																	
Shrug																	
Shoulder Hinge																	

Street Light									
Snake Charmer									
Quadrilateral									
Achilles Stretch A									
Passive Straight Leg Raise									
Active Straight Leg Raise									
Passive Bent Leg Raise									
Active Bent Leg Raise									
Side Leg Raise									

COMMENTS AND SELF-ASSESSMENT

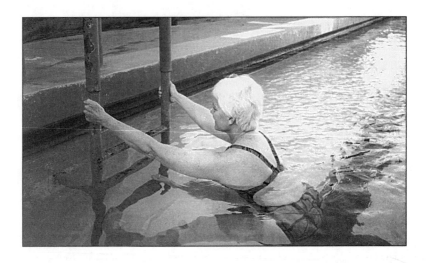

Photograph 7a. Jill beginning Spider-Man. My feet are on the bottom step of the ladder. My back is straight so that all of the hinge is in my hip joints. Notice that my feet are turned slightly pigeon-toed to protect my sacroiliac. My neck, however, is vertical, creating unnecessary strain farther down my spine.

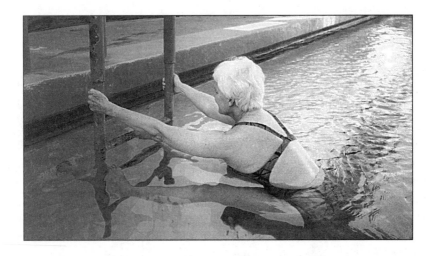

Photograph 7b. Jill, deeper in Spider-Man. After I felt the long muscles in my back and legs release, I was able to move my feet up to a higher step. Notice that I did not move my hands. But I must think about keeping my head and neck in line with my spine.

SECTION I–PLUS:

STANDING AT A WALL IN CHEST-DEEP WATER

A wall provides more stability than a noodle. You can practice all the postures and stretches in the preceding section at the wall, except for Half-Moon, Arch/Slump, and the shoulder stretches that require both arms to participate.

The following additional stretches start from Mountain pose. In these stretches you use the wall as a prop rather than as a stabilizer. You may be able to use the ladder as a bar, for your foot, or as a grab-bar for your hands.

• **Arrow A.** Arrow is horizontal Mountain, based on awareness that there is no "up" or "down" when you are submerged in water. An arrow glides, narrow and straight, without disturbing anything around it. Straight as an arrow is the opposite of slumped and slouchy. Goggles and/or snorkel may be useful if you put your face under water.
1. Stand with your back to the wall.
2. Inhale deeply and hold your breath as you drop your head forward into the water. At the same time bend your knees and lift your feet behind you.
3. Breathing slowly and constantly out through your nose, stretch your arms above your head as far as possible as you push gently off the wall, just below the surface of the water, maintaining your horizontal position. Your face will be down. Point your toes. Align your body as in Mountain.
4. Visualize opening the space between each vertebra and joint just as you did in vertical Mountain. Feel yourself as long as possible, as straight as possible, like an arrow.
5. To return to Mountain, curve your hips forward and bring your feet to the bottom as your raise your head.
6. As an intensification of this stretch, if you have plenty of room, if there is no one in the way, if your back is strong, and if you feel confident, you can push off HARD from the wall. Feel the arrow shoot through the water! The longer and straighter your body is, the farther you will glide. This is what competitive swimmers call "streamlining."

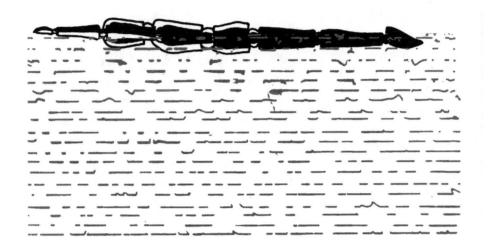

Illustration 30. Arrow.

• **Arrow B.** This is the same as Arrow A except that instead of pushing off from a wall, your hands anchor you to the wall, and a float keeps your feet from sinking. You can practice this posture on your back so that you can breathe constantly, or you can hold your breath and practice it on your stomach.

1. Gripping the wall with one hand, wedge a noodle (or "pull-buoy") between your thighs with the other. Its buoyancy will bring your hips to the surface.
2. Gripping the wall with both hands, float extended out horizontally, long and narrow, like an arrow.
3. Stretch your arms above your head to open your shoulders. Lengthen your spine, opening the space between each vertebra and joint, maintaining your horizontal Mountain pose.
4. Alternately point your toes and flex your ankles if you like.
5. To come out of Arrow B release the noodle, raise your head and drop your feet to the bottom.

BACK STRETCHES AT A WALL

• **Cautious Back-Bend.** I call this stretch "cautious" because you have complete control of it, and because it can be quite minimal if necessary.

1. Facing the wall, hold on to the edge, and stand at arms length away from it.
2. Slowly move your hips and torso toward the wall to create a backward arch. Hold.
3. You may intensify the arch if you feel your spine relax. Do not over-do.
4. Return to Mountain.

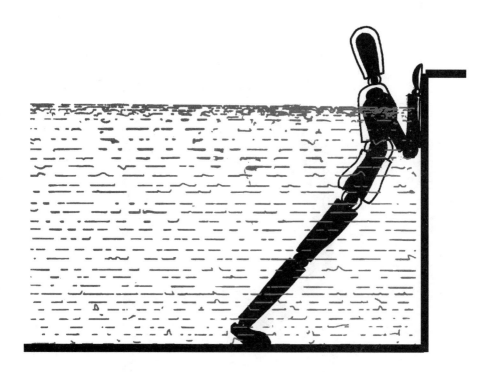

Illustration 31. Cautious Back–Bend

• **Daring Back-Bend.** This stretch is only for the very confident. It can induce flexibility in the upper back as well as the lower back. You must have something secure to hold onto at the edge, like a pipe or ladder. You may find it easier to start with your knees and hip joints bent.

1. Stand with your feet close to the wall, facing away from it, and raising your arms over your head and looking upward, grasp the pipe or ladder.
2. Slowly move your hips and torso away from the wall to create a backward arch. Hold.
3. You may intensify the arch if you feel your spine relax. Do not overdo.
4. Reverse the first steps to return to Mountain.

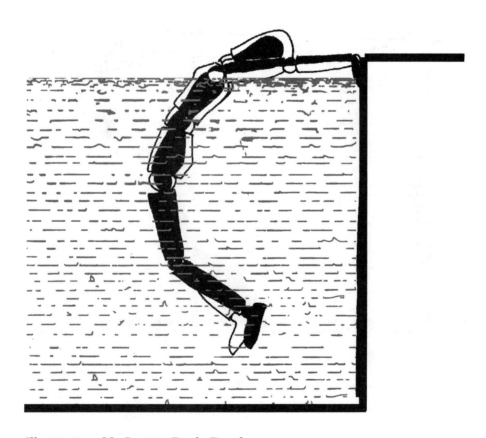

Illustration 32. Daring Back–Bend

- **Cat on a Wall.** You must be able to hold on firmly to the edge of the wall.
1. Facing the wall, hold on to the edge and bring your knees up so that your thighs are perpendicular to the wall.
2. Slowly arch your back, creating backward arch as far as is comfortable. Hold and release.
3. Slowly curve your back forward as far as is comfortable. Hold and release.
4. Repeat, being aware of all the muscles that do this work, and their relation to your pelvis and hip joints.

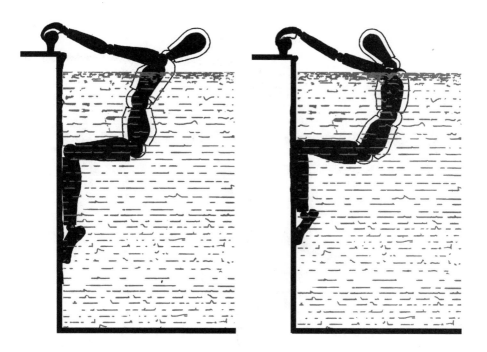

Illustration 33. Cat on a Wall.

- **Hip Swings.**
1. Facing away from the wall, spread your arms out and grip the top of the wall to stabilize yourself.
2. Lift your knees in front of you so that they are free of the bottom.
3. Keeping your back flat and just free of the wall, swing your torso and hips slowly to your right. Hold.
4. Release and repeat to the left.
5. As a gentle movement, you may set up a pendulum motion from side to side.

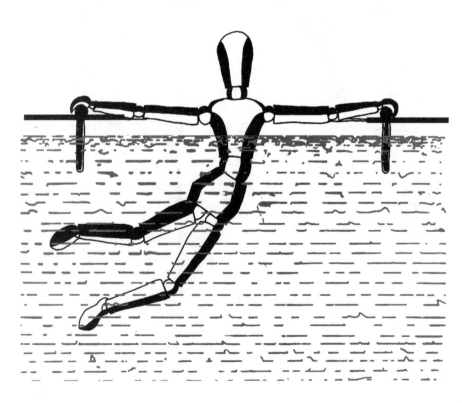

Illustration 34. Hip Swings

HIP OPENERS AT A WALL

• **Standing Triangle.**
1. Face the wall in Mountain with your hands on the edge to stabilize yourself, and your whole body as close to the wall as possible, even touching at your chest, pelvis and knees.
2. Keeping your back erect and your pelvis centered, spread your feet as far apart as you comfortably can.
3. Rotate your thighs outward, knees straight, feet working toward becoming parallel to the wall. Think of your body as pressed between a pane of glass and the wall. Hold. Note that the shallower the water, the more the weight of your body will intensify this posture.
4. Return to Mountain.

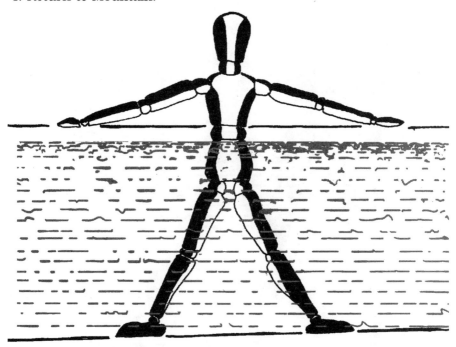

Illustration 35. Standing Triangle

- **High-Step.**
1. Face the wall, holding on to it with both hands, arms straight.
2. Raise or lift your right foot as high as you comfortably can and plant your toes against the wall.
3. Press your body toward the wall so that your right knee bends as far as possible into your chest and your right ankle and toes bend as much as possible. Hold.
4. Return to Mountain. Repeat with left knee.

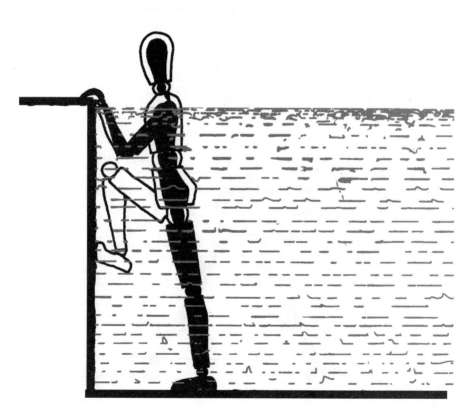

Illustration 36. High–Step

- **Spider-Man.** This can be a very intense stretch, and very satisfying. You must be able to hold on *securely* to the edge of the wall, a ladder, or other grab-bar.
1. Facing the wall, grasp the edge with both hands, arms straight in front of you at shoulder width apart.
2. Keeping your back straight at all times, raise both legs to the wall, as far apart as you can, with your knees straight. Keep your back straight to avoid risk of strain to the lumbar vertebrae.
3. Turn your feet slightly inward, pigeon-toed.
4. Hold, feeling the stretch in your groins.
5. If you feel the groin muscles let go, you may intensify the stretch by raising your feet a little farther on the wall, or separating them a little more. Hold.
6. Return to Mountain.

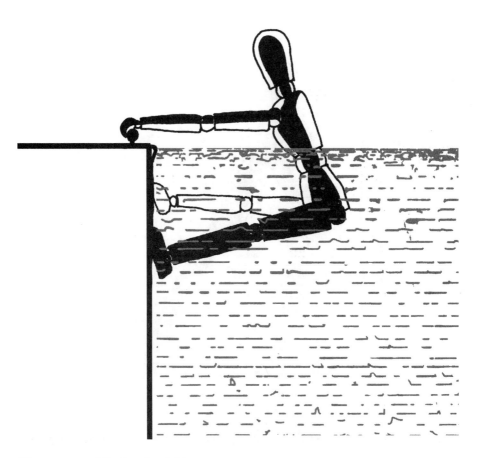

Illustration 37. Spider–Man

LEG STRETCHES AT A WALL

- **Achilles Stretch B.**
1. Face the wall, your feet a couple of feet away from it, and your hands gripping the edge.
2. Pull your shoulders toward the wall, keeping your whole body straight and your heels on the bottom. Feel the stretch in your Achilles tendons, which run down the backs of your ankles.
3. Adjust your distance from the wall to maximize the stretch. Hold.
4. Return to Mountain.

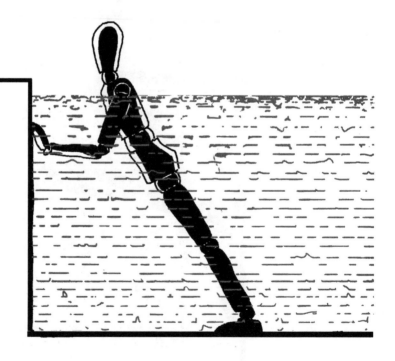

Illustration 38. Achilles B

- **Spring-Board.** This stretch mirrors the vaulting step of a spring-board diver.
1. Face away from the wall, holding on to it with your arms out-stretched.
2. Keeping your back flat against the wall, raise your right knee, bending it so that your lower leg remains parallel to the wall.
3. Hold and return to Mountain.
4. Repeat with your left leg.
5. For a more intense stretch and some abdominal toning, lift both legs at the same time.

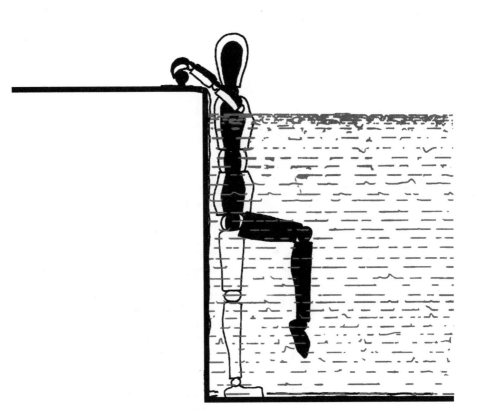

Illustration 39. Spring–Board

STRAIGHT LEG RAISES AT A WALL

Straight leg raises are good for your hips as well as your legs. Remember that flexibility in the hips saves your back from overwork.

- **Goose-Step.** This stretch will also strengthen your abdominal muscles.
1. Face away from a wall, holding on to it with your hands to stabilize yourself.
2. Keeping your back flat against the wall and your pelvis level and centered, raise your right leg straight out in front.
3. Hold and return to Mountain.
4. Repeat with your left leg.
5. For a more intense abdominal involvement, raise both legs at the same time.

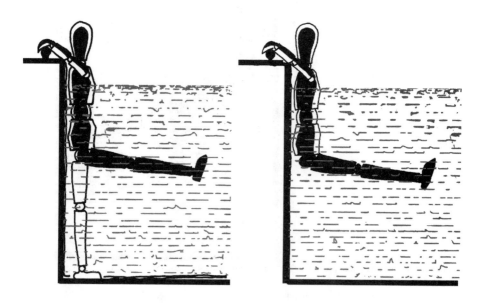

Illustration 40. Goose–Step. One Leg and Two Legs

• **Side Leg Raise at a Wall.** Use a step or ladder or pool-deck of the right height for a ballet bar. Improvise if you need to. Keep your back straight and your pelvis level and centered. Raise your leg no higher than you comfortably can without changing your posture.

1. Standing with the bar to your right, raise your right leg to the side and straighten it and rest your ankle on the bar. Be conscious of your right hip being no higher than your left hip.
2. Rotate your right thigh backward. Hold.
3. Return to Mountain.
4. Repeat with your left leg.
5. For a more intense stretch, you may alternately flex and extend your feet.

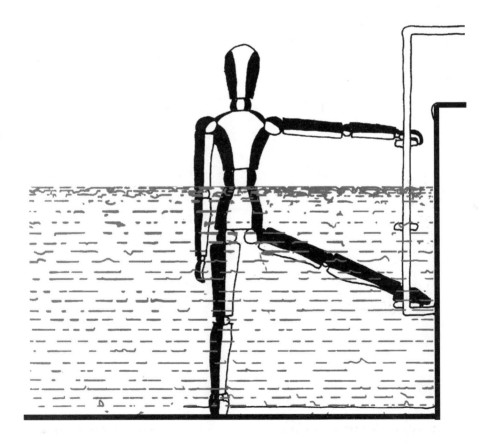

Illustration 41. Side Leg Raise at a Wall

- **Front Leg Raise at a Wall.** Use a step or ladder or pool-deck of the right height for a ballet bar. Improvise if you need to. Keep your back straight and your pelvis level and centered. Raise your leg no higher than you comfortably can without changing your posture.
1. Facing the bar, raise your right leg to the front and straighten it, resting your ankle on the bar. Be conscious of your right hip being no higher than your left hip. Hold.
2. Return to Mountain.
3. For a more intense stretch, you may alternately flex and extend your right foot.

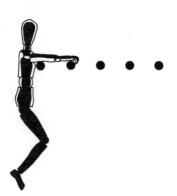

SECTION II. SUSPENDED ON NOODLES IN WATER

AT LEAST CHEST-DEEP

The following stretches require water that is at least chest deep: deep enough that when you bend your knees in a relaxed way they are free of the bottom.

SUSPENDED ZEN: THE STARTING POSTURE

A WaterYoga pose that I call Suspended Zen is the starting pose for stretches you do while suspending your body from a noodle. The most important thing to remember in Suspended Zen is to keep your spine straight and vertical. Don't let your buttocks float up behind you. Don't let your hips float forward. I call this posture Zen because it has the flavor of "sitting Zen" in which the upper body posture is erect but the hips and legs are bent.

- **Suspended Zen**
1. Suspend your body from a noodle. Lean on it as if it were the back fence. Or treat it like an inner tube. Adjust it so that your shoulders and your ears lie on the "plumb line," an imaginary line that runs from the top of your head down through the middle of your torso. The plumb line should be on your axis of gravity. Use a second noodle as a stabilizer, if you want. Float it in front of you parallel to the first noodle, and lightly rest your hands on it, with your arms straight but relaxed.
2. Consciously relax your shoulders. Your scapulae do not strain toward your spine or up toward your ears, but slide down your back. Broaden your shoulders outward, toward a real or imaginary horizon on each side of you. Visualize the spaces in the shoulder joints opening up.
3. Lift the top of your sternum high. This opens up the top of your rib cage. Sense the separateness of your thorax (chest) from your shoulder girdle.
4. Even though your shoulders are resting on the noodle, drop the tips of your shoulders so that your clavicles are as horizontal as possible.
5. Feel the top (actually the back part of the top) of your head rise as if lifted by a balloon. Your chin should not jut out. Tuck it in, without constricting your throat. Feel that your neck seems to elongate as your head rises.
6. Feel, but do not force, the strength in your abdomen. Use it to help lift up your diaphragm.
7. Maintain the natural curve of your spine. If your upper spine tends to be rounded (dowager's hump), use the muscles in your upper back to push the backs of your upper ribs forward. If your lower back curves too much (lordosis), pull your abdomen back toward your spine and tighten your buttocks.
8. Keep your legs relaxed and free, bent at the knees just enough to keep your feet off the bottom.
9. Breathe normally, sensing how similar this posture is to Mountain.

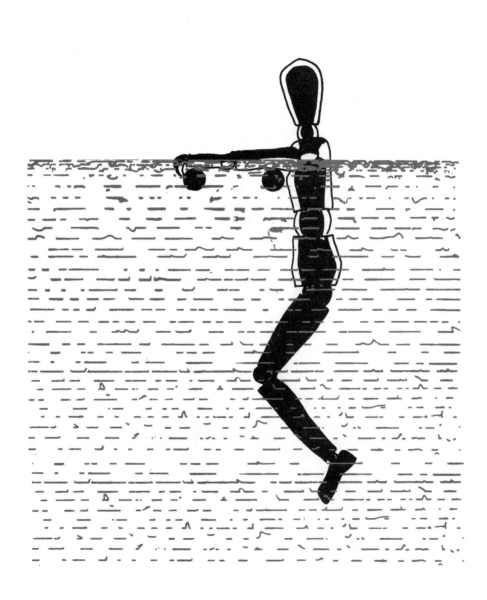

Illustration 42. Suspended Zen

BACK STRETCHES FROM SUSPENDED ZEN

Do all back stretches with your body posture in proper alignment, with your spine in a correct natural curve and with your shoulders relaxed on the noodle.

- **Cat on a Noodle.**
1. Bring your knees up to perpendicular to your body, allowing your lower legs to hang freely, as if you were sitting in a chair.
2. Slowly arch your back, creating lordosis, as far is comfortable. Hold and release.
3. Slowly curve your back forward as far as is comfortable. Hold and release.
4. Repeat, being aware of all the muscles that do this work, and their relation to your pelvis.

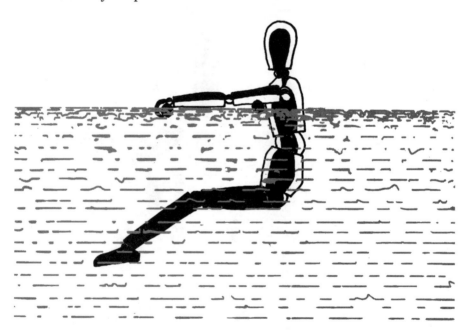

Illustration 43. This is the first phase of Cat on a Noodle and of Pendulum Front to Back.

- **Pendulum Front to Back.**
1. Slowly swing your legs forward, knees bent, feeling your spine curve forward, feeling your abdominal muscles at work. Hold and return to Suspended Zen.
2. Slowly swing your legs back behind you, straightening them if you like, feeling your back arch, feeling your spinal muscles at work. Hold and return to Suspended Zen.
3. Repeat this cycle as if you were a pendulum, if you like.

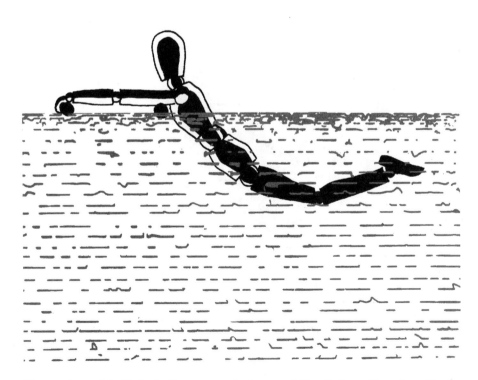

Illustration 44. This is the second phase of Pendulum Front to Back. See Cat on a Wall for the second phase of Cat on a Noodle.

- **Pendulum Side to Side.**

1. Slowly swing your legs, knees bent, to the right, feeling the muscles down the right side of your body at work. Hold and return to Suspended Zen.
2. Repeat on the left.
3. Repeat this cycle as if you were a pendulum, if you like.
4. As an intensification, try to straighten the leg on the "inside of the curve." You will feel the muscles working harder.

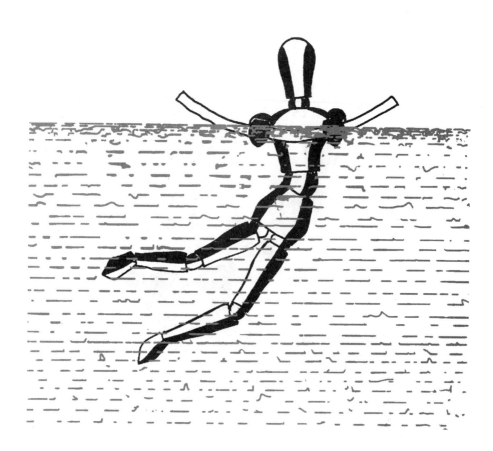

Illustration 45. Pendulum Side to Side

- **Twist, Suspended.** In water, there is minimal risk of strain during the Twist because the vertebrae are not compressed.
1. Slowly rotate your hips and knees to the right, allowing your upper body to follow your hips to the right, keeping your shoulders stable.
2. At the same time, slowly turn your head to the left, keeping your shoulders stable. They are the axis around which your body pivots. See Neck Stretches for proper technique. Hold.
3. Slowly return to center and repeat, turning your hips and knees to the left and your head to the right.

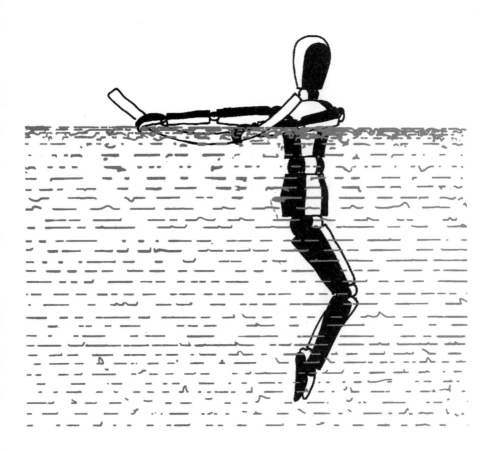

Illustration 46. Twist, Suspended

HIP OPENERS FROM SUSPENDED ZEN

Increased flexibility and strength in hip joints relieves postural strain on the lower back. Keep your spine erect and vertical, neither too curved nor too flat. All movement is in the legs, all stretch in the hips.

• **Arabesque.** This stretch suggests the feeling of flight when a ballet dancer performs an Arabesque. It is also similar to a Chinese movement called "walking with high strides," which is said to dispel emotions like sadness, anger and pensiveness.

1. Very slowly lift one thigh in front of you, and lift the other thigh behind you. Your calves and feet remain relaxed. Visualize yourself doing a "split" as you feel the stretch in the muscles and tendons in your hips. Hold.
2. Very slowly reverse your legs. Hold. Don't move so fast that you bob up and down. Remember that this is a stretch, not a movement.
3. Return to Suspended Zen.

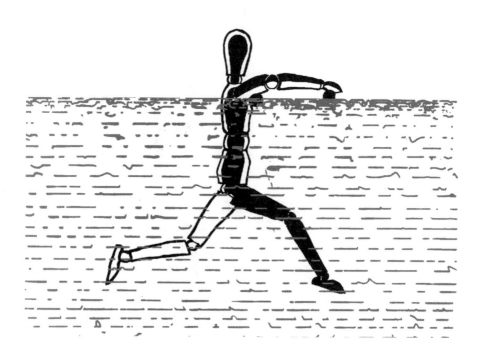

Illustration 47. Arabesque

- **Triangle, Suspended.**
1. Slowly spread your legs out to the sides, straightening your knees, keeping your feet clear of the bottom.
2. Rotate your thighs outward at the hip joints. Hold. Visualize your body pressed front-to-back between two panes of glass. Identify the hip muscles that make the triangle wider.
3. Rotate your ankle joints in slow circles, forward and backward.
4. Return to Suspended Zen.

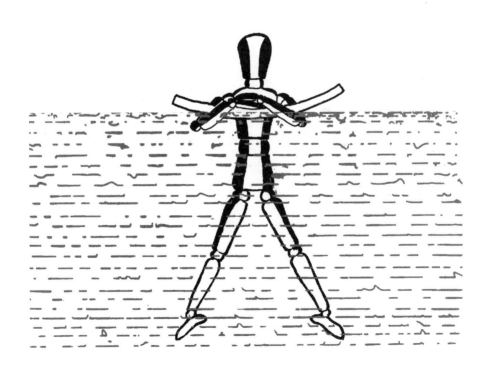

Illustration 48. Triangle, Suspended

- **Diamond, Suspended.**
1. Slowly spread your legs out to the sides, knees bent, feet together and clear of the bottom. Feel the outward rotation of your thighs at the hip joints.
2. Try to press the soles of your feet together. Visualize your body front-to-back pressed between two panes of glass. Hold.
3. Feel the strength of your groin and hip muscles as you make the diamond wider and shorter and flatter.
4. Return to Suspended Zen.

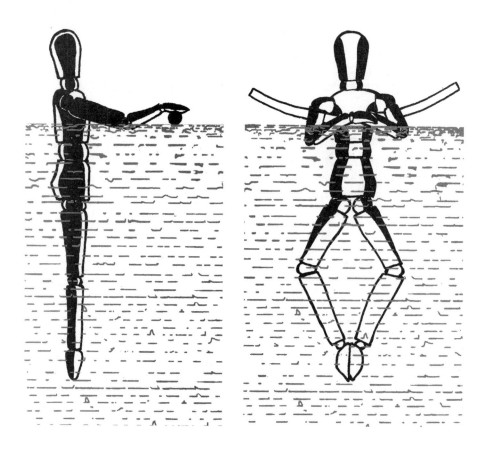

Illustration 49. Diamond, Suspended. Side view

Illustration 50. Diamond, Suspended. Front view

SECTION II-PLUS

GENTLE MOVEMENTS FROM SUSPENDED ZEN

As you become comfortable doing the stretches of Suspended Zen, and understand how your body interacts with the water, you may want to explore some gentle movements. The following are my favorites. Practice them with the grace and rhythm of dancing.

• **Swing to Sides.** This is an intensification of Pendulum: Side to Side. It starts just below your shoulders. It works all of the muscles of your torso, massages your organs, and energizes your spine. Keep your shoulders stable on the noodles. Do not let your body twist.
1. Lift your right hips, legs and feet to the right side as far as you can.
2. Let them drop, and use their momentum to continue the swing to the left side.
3. Lift your left hips, legs and feet to the left side as far as you can.
4. Repeat rhythmically following the flow of your body's momentum against the resistance of the water.

• **Swing Front to Back.** This is an intensification of Pendulum: Front to Back. The principles are the same as Swing to Sides, but you may choose to involve your legs more.

1. Keeping your legs softly together at all times, bring your knees toward the surface in front of you. You may round your back, or not.
2. Let your knees and feet drop, and use their momentum to continue the swing behind you.
3. Lift your legs toward the surface behind you and extend your feet as far behind you as you feel comfortable. You may let your buttocks rise toward the surface. You may arch your back or not.
4. Repeat rhythmically, following the flow of your body's momentum against the resistance of the water.

• **Bicycle.** Many people today do "aqua-jogging" while wearing a flotation belt. I do not feel comfortable in a flotation belt. Bicycling while suspended from a noodle gives me a better feeling because my back hangs free. Bicycle is an intensification of Arabesque.

1. Keeping your back vertical, and taking care not to twist, make your feet and legs trace the action of leisurely pedaling a bicycle.

- **Sit-Ups, Suspended.** This is a true exercise, an effective abdominal toner. Keep your back straight!
1. Keeping your back straight, raise both legs in front of you, straightening them as soon as you are clear of the bottom. If your abdominal muscles are very strong, you can bring your feet all the way to the surface.
2. You may intensify the movement by pointing your toes, or by flexing your ankles.
3. Let your feet and knees drop, and use their momentum (inertia) to return to Suspended Zen.
4. Repeat rhythmically, following the flow of your body's motion against the resistance of the water.

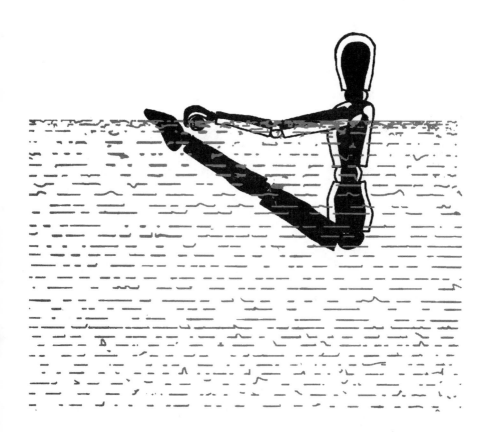

Illustration 51. Sit–Ups, Suspended

DIARY OF WATERYOGA PRACTICE
SECOND LIST: AT A WALL AND IN SUSPENDED ZEN

PRACTICE DATE												
Arrow A												
Arrow B												
Suspended Zen												
Cautious Back-Bend												
Daring Back-Bend												
Cat on a Wall												
Hip Swings												
Standing Triangle												
High Step												
Spider-Man												
Achilles Stretch B												
Spring-Board												
Goose-Step												
Side Leg Raise at a Wall												
Front Leg Raise at a Wall												
Cat on a Noodle												
Pendulum Front to Back												
Pendulum Side to Side												
Twist, Suspended												

Arabesque							
Triangle, Suspended							
Diamond, Suspended							
Swing to Sides							
Swing Front to Back							
Bicycle							
Sit-ups, Suspended							

COMMENTS AND SELF-ASSESSMENT

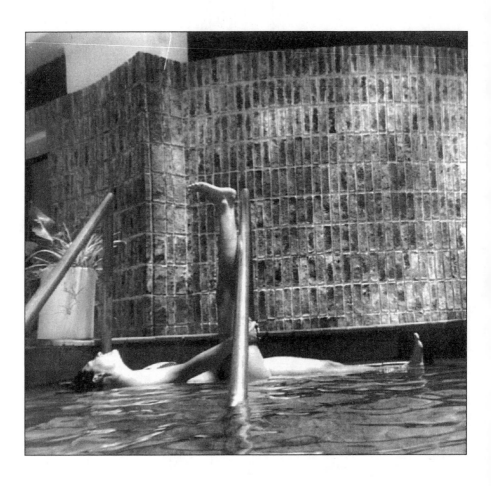

Photograph 8. Cecelia in Straight Leg Raise, Reclining. She is lying on the top step of a warm salt water pool at an elegant spa in Uruguay. She will relax her neck when she relaxes into the stretch.

SECTION III. IN SHALLOW WATER

The following stretches are guides only. I include them so that you will see how you can adapt WaterYoga to your back yard pool, hot tub, whirlpool, or any shallow water, even your bathtub. Adaptability of the stretches will depend on your height, depth of the water, and how large a space you have.

I developed the following shallow water stretches in the warm water off a sandy beach at Montevideo, Uruguay. Slight waves interfered with my balance. The water was salty, of course, which greatly increased my buoyancy. The stretches will feel a little different in the lesser buoyancy of fresh water. I stayed in the water a long time, and was very glad I had sun protection.

KNEELING IN WATER UP TO YOUR CHEST

In water that is up to your chest when you are kneeling on the bottom you can practice **Arrow Posture**, and **Neck, Shoulder, Ankle, Foot,** and **Hand Stretches.** Start as in Mountain, but kneeling on the bottom. Use a noodle for stabilization if you need to. Review WATERYOGA STRETCHES FROM MOUNTAIN POSE for descriptions. You can also adapt the following stretches:

HIP OPENERS
- **Five Pointed Star, Kneeling**
- **Pelvis Rock, Kneeling**
- **Stork, Kneeling**
- **Triangle, Kneeling**
- **Leg Raises**

BACK STRETCHES.
- **Arch/Slump, Kneeling**
- **Twist, Kneeling**

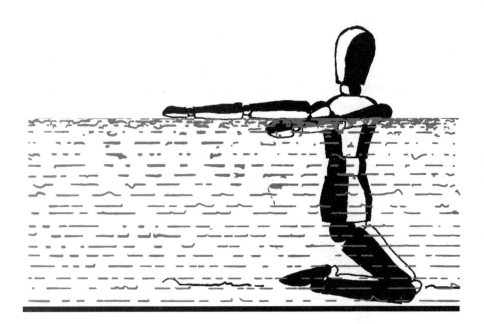

Illustration 52. Twist, Kneeling

- **Triangle Split.** This is a classic yoga pose. You will still be standing in the finished stretch.
1. Stand in Mountain and move to Triangle. The water level should be about at your waist at this point.
2. Rotate your right foot 90 degrees to the right, and continue the rotation into the thigh and hip joint.
3. Rotate your left foot about 10 degrees to the right. At the same time rotate your left hip to the left, keeping your left leg active (knee straight but not hyperextended and knee-cap up).
4. Extend both arms straight out to your sides.
5. Keeping your back erect, bend your right knee so that your torso drops down. Do not allow your right shin to pass beyond vertical, directly over your right ankle. Instead, to deepen the stretch, move your right foot away from your body. Your shoulders remain horizontal throughout, as do your extended arms. Hold.
6. Return to Standing Triangle and repeat to the left side.

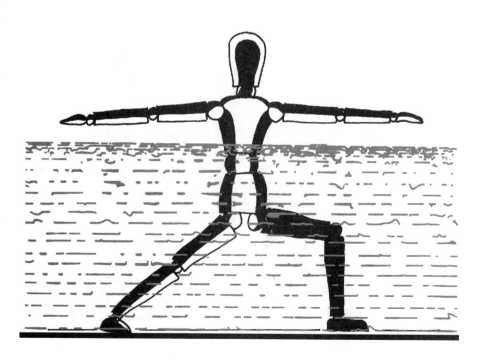

Illustration 53. Triangle Split

• **Warrior.** This is a classic yoga pose. I don't know why it is called "Warrior," but it is especially useful for toning the psoas muscles. You will still be standing on your feet in the finished stretch.

1. Stand in Mountain and move to Triangle. The water should be about at your waist at this point.
2. Rotate your right foot 90 degrees to the right, and continue the rotation into the thigh and hip joint.
3. At the same time, rotate your left foot about 45 degrees to the right, keeping your left leg active (knee straight but not hyperextended and knee-cap up).
4. Take some time to check your body alignment. Steps two and three mean that your torso remains erect and faces evenly to the right. Both arms remain at your sides. Feel the pull in your pelvis and make sure that it is level.

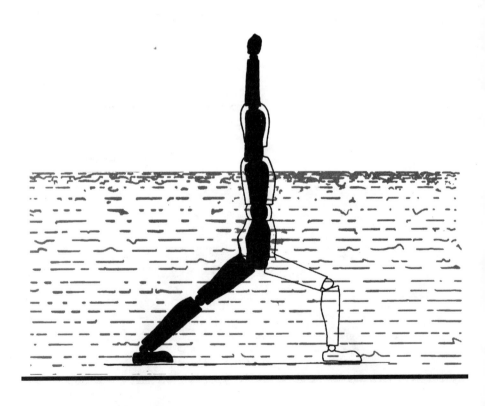

Illustration 54. Warrior

5. Keeping your back erect, bend your right knee so that your torso drops straight down. Do not allow your right shin to pass beyond vertical, directly over your right ankle. Instead, to deepen the stretch, move your left foot back away from your body. Hold.
6. Return to Triangle and repeat to the left side.
7. To intensify this stretch, repeat steps 1 through 5, then raise both arms straight up, hands facing each other. Look toward the sky.

• **T'ai Ch'i.** This is a standing posture. You will still be standing on your feet in the finished stretch.
1. Stand with your feet at hip width apart. Turn your toes slightly in.
2. Bend your knees, ankles and hips to about 45 degrees. Hold. Some teachers suggest that this posture can be held for minutes rather than seconds!
3. Return to Mountain.

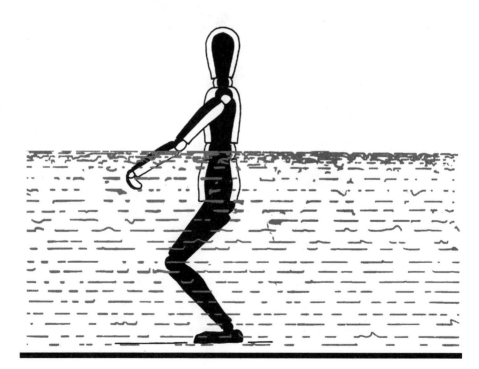

Illustration 55. T'ai Ch'i

• **Hip Press.** This is a standing stretch. You will still be standing on your feet in the finished stretch.

1. Stand with your feet at hip width apart. Turn your toes slightly in.
2. Bending forward at the hip joints, place your hands on your hip joints, fingers down.
3. Press the tops of your femurs toward your back. Visualize your pelvis moving forward at the same time.
4. Return to Mountain.

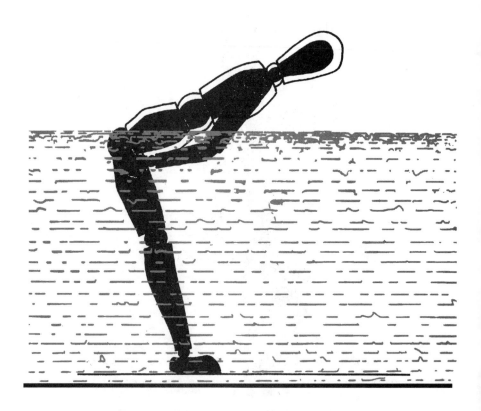

Illustration 56. Hip Press

• **Half-Yoga-Sit.** This is an advanced yoga posture on land but it should be easier in kneeling depth in water. A noodle may help you to stabilize yourself.

1. As you squat down to submerge your body up to your chest, place your right ankle on your left knee. Keep your back straight and your shoulders relaxed.
2. In the finished posture, you are balanced on your left toes, with your left buttock resting on your left ankle. Hold.
3. Rise up, or float out.
4. Repeat, placing your left ankle on your right knee.

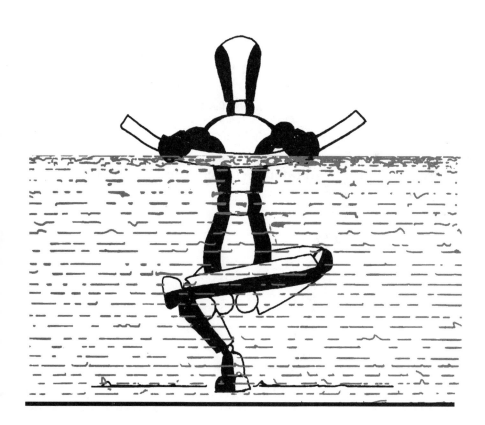

Illustration 57. Half-Yoga Sit

SITTING IN WATER UP TO TO YOUR CHEST

In water that is up to your chest when you are sitting on the bottom you can do Arrow Posture and most **Neck, Shoulder, Ankle, Foot,** and **Hand Stretches**. In addition, you may adapt the following stretches:

• **Triangle, Kneeling.** Kneel on the leg that is to the rear.

• **Half-Yoga-Sit.** You must be able to support additional upper body weight.

Try the following additional stretches in sitting-depth water.

• **Ankle-Sit.** This is a basic yoga pose for stretching the ankles, and for meditation. It is a good posture for doing shoulder stretches if the water level is right.

1. Start from a kneeling position. Extend your toes back behind you. Keeping your back straight, let your buttocks settle onto your heels. Hold. Some people can comfortably hold this posture indefinitely.

2. In an intensification of this stretch, place your knees and ankles far enough apart so that your buttocks can settle between them.

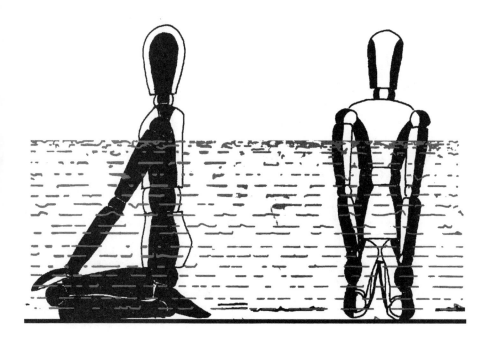

Illustration 58. Ankle-Sit. Side and front views

• **Tailor's Seat A.** This is the way you may have sat as a child. If you can't do it any more, this might be the time to relearn it. You may sit on the edge of a brick or other support to make it easier.

1. Keeping your back straight, sit cross-legged with your hands on your knees. Hold.
2. Still keeping your back straight, drop your torso forward over your legs. Hold.
3. Release.
4. You may intensify this stretch by gently pulling against your knees with your hands as you drop your torso forward.

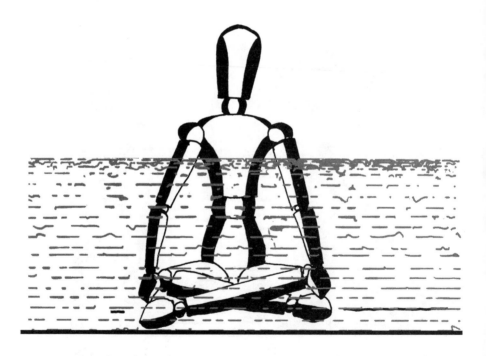

Illustration 59. Tailor's seat A

Cat. Do this traditional yoga stretch if the water level allows you to be on your hands and knees and keep your back submerged and your head above water when you need to breathe. Warm your back well before you start.

1. From a position on your hands and knees, raise your back like a cat hissing at a dog, and at the same time lower your head so that your chin is on your chest. Hold.
2. Return to the straight-back position.
3. Drop your back so that your spine is sway-backed like that of an old horse, and at the same time raise your head so that your chin is in the air. Hold.
4. Return to the straight-backed position.
5. Slowly repeat the cycle.

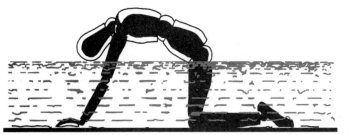

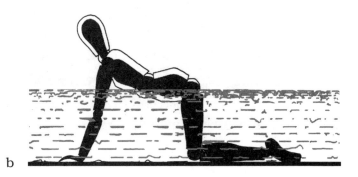

Illustration 60. Cat. View a shows the back extended. View b shows the back arched. (This is confusing because the cat "arches" its back oppositely from us humans.)

• **Tailor's Seat B.** Keep your back straight throughout so that the stretch is in your hips. Some people find this stretch very easy. I am one of those others who find it impossible.

1. Sit with both legs straight out in front, putting your torso and thighs at an aproximate right angle.
2. Keeping your feet flat on the bottom, bend both knees and let them fall out to the sides as you move your feet past each other, your left lower leg closer to your body than your right. Support your upper body with one hand if necessary.
3. Pick up your right ankle with one or two hands and place it on top of your left knee, creating an equilateral triangle of your two thighs and the stack of your two lower legs. Don't be discouraged if your left knee won't stay on the bottom and your right knee is high above your left knee. Hold.
4. Release and repeat with the left ankle.

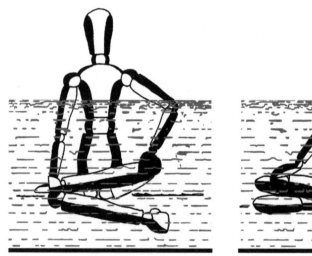
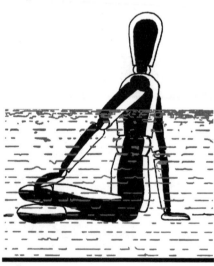

Illustration 61. Tailor's Seat B. Front and side views

IN VERY SHALLOW WATER

In less than a foot of water, and if you have enough space, you can practice **Arrow Posture** and many stretches. Just be sure there is enough water to cover and warm your hip joints. Because the bottom absorbs the heat of the sun, very shallow open water can be warmer than deep water. It is all right if some parts of your body touch bottom as long as you maintain correct body alignment.

You can do some stretches in a bathtub or baby pool. Use a mat to do stretches if the bottom is a hard surface.

As long as your head is out of the water enough for you to breathe normally, you can experiment with **Mountain** and **Suspended Zen** stretches in a horizontal position. You can also practice the following stretches:

• **Ankle, Foot, Hand Stretches**

• **Ankle-Sit,** if you are comfortable with substantial added body-weight

• **Tailor's Seat A**

• **Tailor's Seat B**

The following stretches are especially suited to very shallow water.

• Hip Hinges.
1. Sit with your legs straight out in front. Support your upper body with your hands if necessary. Hold.
2. Spread your legs as far apart as possible. Hold.
3. Bend forward, using your hip joints as a hinge. Do not hump your back. Hold.
4. Return to 2.
5. Place your right foot (especially the heel) in your left groin (not under it).
6. Adjust your hips so that your torso faces your left leg.
7. Bend forward over your left knee, using your hip joints as a hinge. Do not hump your back. Hold.
8. Straighten up and repeat steps 5 through 7 over your right leg.

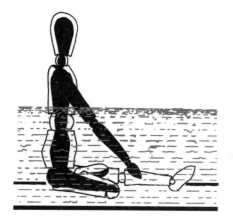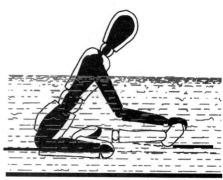

Illustration 62. Hip Hinges

- **Cobra.** This is a favorite traditional yoga posture for back flexibility and strength. It is less strenuous in water than on land.
1. Start on your hands and knees. Extend your toes behind you. Keep your arms straight as you walk your hands toward your head, allowing your hips to drop to the bottom
2. Raise your chin. Hold. Feel the arch in your back. Keep your shoulders low and wide.
3. Return to hands and knees.

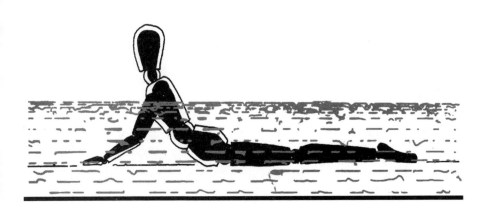

Illustration 63. Cobra

For stretches in which you are lying in very shallow water, start in Arrow, lying on your back. Put something under your head to keep your nose above water, if needed. It should not be so thick that it distorts your posture. Keep your back straight throughout. Bend only in the hinge of your hip joints.

• **Alexander-Style Relaxation.** This posture is adapted from a relaxation method that is taught in the Alexander Technique. You can do it before and/or after your stretches.
1. Lie on your back with a small pad under your head to remove any strain from your neck.
2. Slide both feet toward your head so that your knees are up and bent at a right angle while your feet rest flat on the bottom.
3. Widen your shoulders, and angling your elbows away from your body, rest your hands on your chest.
4. Lengthen your spine. As it relaxes, you may want to slide your pelvis toward your feet.
5. Find the balance in which your legs remain vertical without muscular assistance.
6. Rest. That's all there is to this very relaxing posture.

• Leg Raise to Side, Reclining

1. Lie on your right side, propping your head up on your right hand and elbow.
2. Keeping your left leg straight, raise it up no more than 45 degrees. Hold.
3. Lower your left leg and repeat, lying on your left side and raising your right leg.

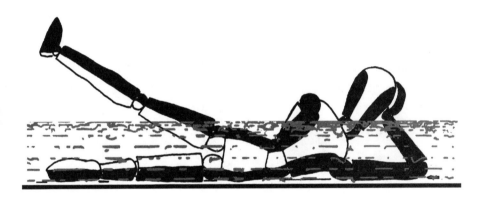

Illustration 64. Leg Raise to Side, Reclining. View from back

• **Straight Leg Raise, Reclining.** Use a noodle in this stretch. Keep your back straight and your neck relaxed.

1. Lie on your back.
2. Keeping your right leg straight and active (knee cap raised and foot flexed), raise it up as close to right angles with your body as is comfortable. Feel your hip act as a hinge. Keep your left leg active, but straight and flat on the bottom.
3. Loop a noodle over the arch of your flexed foot and hold it with both hands to pull your leg a little farther into the stretch. Hold.
4. Release the noodle and return to Arrow.
5. Repeat, raising the left leg.
6. As an intensification of this stretch, raise both legs at once.

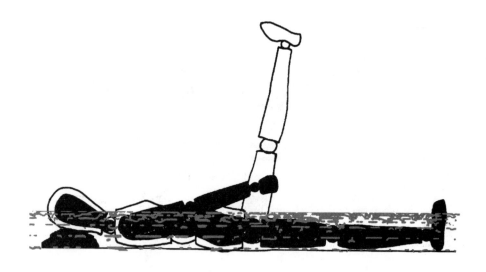

Illustration 65. Straight Leg Raise, Reclining

• **Knee Hug.**

1. Lying on your back in Arrow, raise both knees to your chest, while keeping your spine straight. Do not arch or hump your back. Keep your chin and your neck relaxed.
2. Put your arms around your legs and draw them as tight to your body as comfortable. Hold.
3. Return to Arrow.
4. As an intensification of this stretch, raise each knee separately to your chest, while keeping the other leg active, but straight and flat on the bottom.
5. As a further intensification, flex, extend and rotate the ankle of the straight leg and then the bent leg.

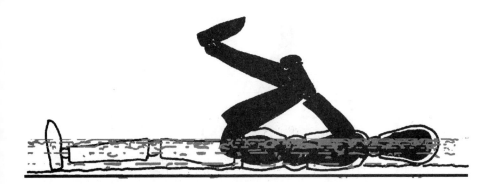

Illustration 66. Knee Hug

• **Straight Leg Twist, Reclining.** Your arms and shoulders will remain stable throughout this stretch.
1. Lying on your back, extend both arms out to the sides.
2. Shift your pelvis so its weight rests on your right hip.
3. Raise your straight left leg up, and swing it over to your right and let it drop as close to your right hand as possible. At the same time, let your head turn toward your left. Hold.
4. Return to Arrow and repeat, twisting to the left.

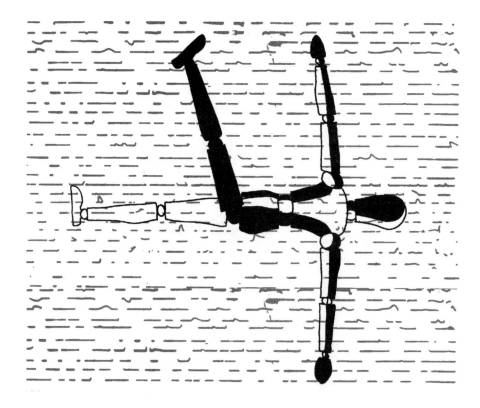

llustration 67. Straight Leg Twist, Reclining. View from above

- **Bent Leg Twist, Reclining.** Your arms and shoulders will remain stable throughout this stretch.
1. Lying on your back, extend both arms out to the sides.
2. Slide your left foot toward your head to bring your knee up and bent at a right angle while your let foot remains flat on the bottom.
3. Shift your pelvis so its weight rests on your right hip as you swing your left knee to the right as far as you can. At the finish your left lower leg is parallel to your right leg and to the right of it. At the same time, let your head turn toward your left. Hold.
4. Return to Arrow and repeat, twisting to the left.
5. As an intensification of this stretch, slide both feet toward your head so that both knees are up, and holding the knees and ankles together, twist to the right and repeat to the left.

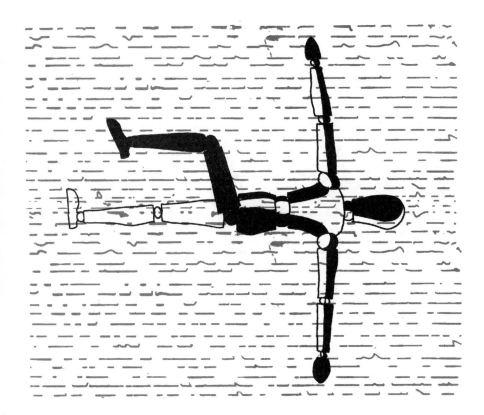

Illustration 68.Bent Leg Twist, Reclining. View from above.

• Crossed Knee (Mild)

1. Start in Alexander-Style Relaxation posture.
2. Place your right ankle on your left thigh.
3. Place your right hand on your right knee to push it lightly away from you. Do not let your pelvis shift. Hold.
4. Release and repeat with your left ankle on your right thigh.
5. Return to Arrow.
6. As an intensification of this stretch, reach through the triangle of your thighs and one calf and grasp the other calf, lacing your fingers together.
7. Pull your calf toward your head. Hold.
8. Release. Reverse your legs and repeat.

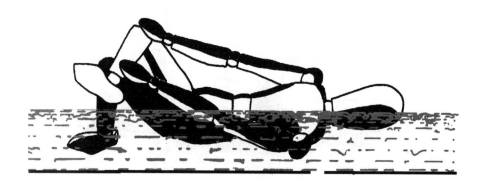

llustration 69. Crossed Knee (Mild). Right ankle rests on left knee.

• Crossed Knee (Strong)

1. Start in Crossed Knee (Mild).
2. Clasp your hands around your left calf or knee. You may have to raise your upper torso temporarily in order to do this.
3. Pull your left leg toward your chest. Hold.
4. Release. Reverse your legs and repeat.

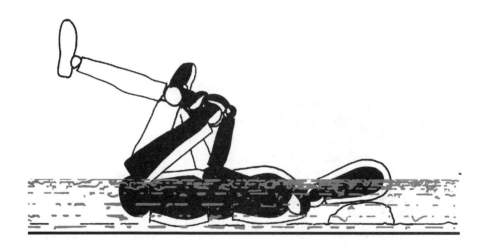

Illustration 70. Crossed Knee (Strong). Left ankle rests on right knee.

SECTION IV
IN WARM WATER ANYWHERE

To practice the stretches in this section, all you need to do is submerge the body part to be stretched in warm water for several minutes until it is warm and relaxed. Here, you can use the tub, sink or wash-basin. If the water is deep, use a noodle for flotation if necessary.

• **Foot and Ankle Stretch.** Stretching the feet and ankles improves the circulation to the whole body. Taoists consider the soles of the feet very important, because they are farthest from the center of the body, and yet are an important place where many arteries of the legs meet the veins. In shallow water you could start in Crossed Knee or Alexander-Style Posture.
1. Gently rub the sole and top of the right foot.
2. Pull each toe to its fullest extension and separation.
3. Press your thumbs or fingers into both arches (transverse and longitudinal).
4. Gently twist the end of the foot inward, then outward.
5. Turn the ankle inward and outward.
6. Rotate the ankle clockwise and counterclockwise.
7. Repeat with the left foot and ankle.

• **Wrist and Finger Stretch.** Check with your health care provider before you practice these stretches if you have carpal tunnel syndrome or arthritis.
1. Hold your right elbow against your body.
2. Put your left palm over the back of your right hand and gently pull your right hand down toward your right forearm.
3. Turn your right hand palm up and gently pull it back toward your right forearm with your left hand.
4. Gently pull each finger and thumb to its fullest extension and separation.
5. Repeat for left wrists and fingers.
6. Alternate stretching your fingers wide and making fists.

• **Jaw Stretch.** Check with your dentist if you suspect any problem like TMJ (temporomandibular joint) dysfunction. More people hold their jaw muscles too tensely than let their jaw hang open all the time. Submerge your jaw area in warm water to warm the tissues before you begin.

1. Open your mouth enough to allow your jaws to move freely.
2. Slide your lower jaw forward, moving your lower teeth in front of your upper teeth. Hold. Slide it back to normal again.
3. Slide your lower jaw to the right of your upper jaw. Hold.
4. Slide it back to normal again.
5. Repeat, sliding it to the left.
6. Open your jaws wide. Hold.
7. Close your jaws.
8. Open your lips wide. Move them in every direction. Make faces.
9. Relax your face and jaw.

SECTION V. IN THE SHOWER

You can practice WaterYoga stretches in the shower if you don't mind using up all the hot water. It is not, strictly speaking, WaterYoga. This is because the shower does not provide the wonderful benefit of weightlessness.

When I feel stiff or when my back is unstable I can hear my inner voice telling me, "Get under the shower." The hot water itself helps me immensely. But I also think my body is so imprinted from WaterYoga that it responds to the healing suggestion that the shower droplets whisper.

The stretches that you can do are determined by the space you have in your shower, and by its physical layout. Because it is all too easy to slip and fall in a shower, please do WaterYoga in the shower ONLY if your balance is good and you have a grab bar to hold onto. For traction on the floor, use a rubber mat. Face away from the shower head. Adjust the angle so that the shower stream falls at the right level on your back.

Start in **Mountain Posture.**

POSSIBLE STRETCHES FOR THE SHOWER

- **Tree**
- **Stork**
- **Achilles Stretch, A and B**
- **Tai Ch'i**
- **Hip Press**
- **Shoulder, Neck, Ankle, Hand Stretches**
- **Cautious Back Bend**
- **Arch/Slump**
- **Bent Leg Raise**
- **Twist.** Be careful to keep your face away from the shower stream so you won't get water up your nose!

• **Half Dog.** This stretch is called "half-dog" because it is similar to the traditional yoga pose "downward-facing dog." It requires a sturdy shower wall.
1. Stand so that your hands on the shower wall with your arms straight will stabilize your upper body when you hinge your hip joints forward.
2. Lean your whole body forward so that your hands are on the wall, arms straight, fingers up. This is actually a mild Achilles Stretch.
3. Walk your hands down the wall until they are at hip height, keeping your back straight so that your whole body hinges into a right angle at the hip joint. Do not arch your back.
4. Feel the gentle warmth of the water as your shoulder joints open, your clavicles fall to the sides of your rib cage, your thighs pull away from the wall and your spine lengthens. Visualize the dinosaur's tail dragging your buttocks back toward the drain. Remember that this is an image only! If it physically happened, your hands would slide away from the wall and you would fall down. Hold.
5. Return to Mountain.

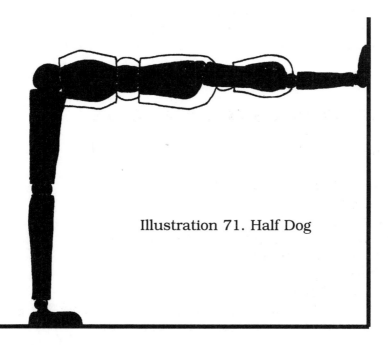

Illustration 71. Half Dog

- **Cat in the Shower**. Do this traditional yoga stretch only if you know you can get down onto the floor and up again with no problem. See Illustration 60.
1. Position the shower stream so that it gently hits your lower back while you kneel on all fours with your back straight. If water falls too high on your back, you may get water up your nose in step 2.
2. Raise your back like a cat hissing at a dog, and at the same time lower your head so that your chin is on your chest. Hold.
3. Return to the straight-back position.
4. Drop your back so that your spine is sway-backed like that of an old horse, and at the same time raise your head so that your chin is in the air. Hold.
5. Return to the straight-backed position.
6. Slowly repeat the cycle.

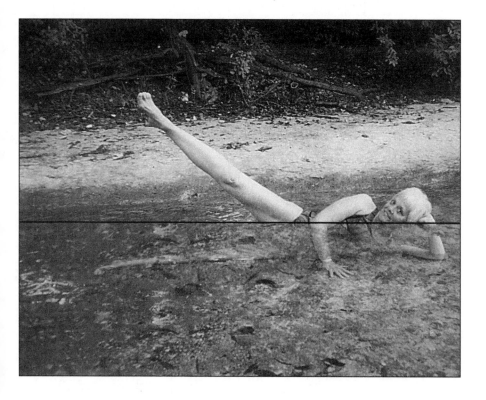

Photograph 9. Jill in Side Leg Raising, Reclining. A horizontal line
show the maximum water depth in which I can comfortably do this
stretch. The locale is a warm sun-lit sandy-bottomed stream. You can
also do this in a wading or baby pool.

DIARY OF WATERYOGA PRACTICE
THIRD LIST: IN SHALLOW WATER

PRACTICE DATE										
Twist, Kneeling										
Triangle Split										
Warrior										
Tai Ch'i										
Hip Press										
Half-Yoga Sit										
Ankle Sit										
Tailor's Seat A										
Cat										
Tailor's Seat B.										
Hip Hinges										
Cobra										
Leg Raise to Side, Reclining										
Straight Leg Raise, Reclining										
Knee Hug										
Straight Leg Twist, Reclining										
Bent Leg Twist, Reclining										
Crossed Knee (Mild)										
Crossed Knee (Strong)										

Foot and Ankle Stretch											
Wrist and Finger Stretch											
Jaw Stretch											
Half Dog											
Cat in the Shower											

COMMENTS AND SELF-ASSESSMENT

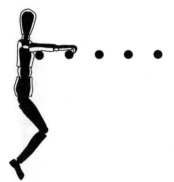

PART FIVE: BACK PAIN AND SPASM—SPECIAL PRACTICE

Incapacitating disability of the back is a common complaint in men and women of all ages. It can strike without warning in inconvenient places and the sufferer cannot be moved at all. The irony of this acute phase is that when you most need a warm pool, you can't get to it.

This part grows from the course of my own WaterYoga practice in dealing with incapacitating back spasm. It is not intended as medical advice, and may not be "what the doctor ordered" for you. Your health care provider is the person to consult about your particular condition.

Back sufferers who compare notes know that no two backs seem to be the same. Practice only the postures and stretches that seem right for you. Ignore the rest. On the other hand, your special back may invite healing stretches that other people would shudder to try. Or the soothing effect of weightlessness in warm water may be enough for you.

Start WaterYoga as soon as you can get to warm water. Start by merely standing in the shower if it helps, but be aware that you won't have an important ingredient: weightlessness. The sooner you feel safe submerging your body in warm water, the sooner the healing process can begin, as the absence of weight-caused compression combined with the warm water invites your spastic muscles to relax. Although nothing may happen for a while, weightlessness and warmth can by themselves bring a soothing respite from pain and spasm.

During the acute phase of a back spasm, do nothing more than support your head with a noodle and let your body relax, free from the compressive weight of your own body on your vertebrae and nerves. It would be reckless to try any postures or stretches because the slightest wrong move could bring on spasm and terrible nerve pain. Your own body will probably tell you that. But you can assist the warm water in achieving its relaxation goal by practicing some of the complementary techniques discussed in Part VI. Remember that the iron grip of a spastic muscle can prevent a displaced vertebrae or bulging disc from returning to normal alignment even in a weightless environment. Although a normal muscle can often relax in about 30 seconds or so, you may have to outwait a spastic muscle for many long, patient days.

During the sub-acute phase, when there is indication that the spasm is abating, it is still important to rest passively for fifteen minutes at least, before attempting any stretches. This will allow the warm water to play its part in softening the tissues. Then you cautiously begin to attempt slight gentle stretches that invite any displaced bones to reseat themselves so that your body can free up pinched nerves.

During several of my back episodes, my spine was visibly and palpably displaced. I have been told that the language of "displaced bones" belongs to osteopathic and chiropractic theory, and is not generally accepted in the medical and physical therapy communities. During two separate WaterYoga practices, however, I felt the physical "shift" in my spine as it actually took place, and each time I knew kinesthetically that I would be "better." My daughter saw the difference in my posture as I left the pool. I could feel the difference in the set of my skeleton with my hand and point with precision to the location of the shift.

(Similar shifts have occurred outside of WaterYoga practice. I recently experienced a totally unexpected shift in a thoracic vertebra and/or its connection to my lower ribs while doing a supported back arch on my bed. My rib cage immediately became measurably smaller.)

Perhaps you will know you are in the sub-acute phase when you can read about the following stretches without wincing. The message in this sentence is, of course: don't push yourself past what your own body tells you you can do. This message is balanced by admonition to follow the advice of the medical professional who is familiar with your problem.

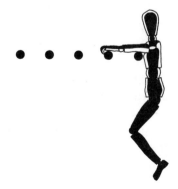

RELAXATION STRETCHES FOR THE LOWER BACK

The following stretches have little or no active component. Their object is to induce a slight movement while the muscles remain completely relaxed. The image I like is the swaying motion of seaweed or marsh grass under water. I hope you have been lucky enough to see marsh grass swaying, using a face mask and snorkel, so that you will be able to think of your back gently swaying.

- **Lengthening the Spine.**
1. Supporting yourself on a noodle, rest passively until your body is warmed and comfortable. This should be at least ten to fifteen minutes. Stabilize yourself by resting your hands on a second noodle, held parallel in front of you, if you like. Review all your muscles to make sure they are relaxed.
2. Let your body respond to its weightlessness in the water. Visualize your vertebrae separating, making room for nerves and discs and muscles, allowing them to heal.
3. Visualize your back lengthening almost imperceptively, but don't do anything. Listen for the message from your back. Wait for its permission before you respond.
4. If your back is ready, very tentatively, gingerly, consciously, allow your back to lengthen. Don't do anything. Just allow it to happen in your mind.
5. Relax. If there were no adverse effects, do it again after a while.

- **Marsh Grass.**
1. Supporting yourself on a noodle, rest passively until your body is warmed and comfortable. Spend at least ten to fifteen minutes. Stabilize yourself by resting your hands on a second noodle, held parallel in front of you, if you like. Review all your muscles to make sure they are relaxed. This may be enough to do in the beginning days.
2. Let your body respond to its weightlessness in the water. Your head is like the top leaves above the surface. Your feet are like the roots, reaching deep but not attached to anything. Your body is the stem, drifting ever so slightly and slowly in the gentle movement of the water.

• **Swaying to the Side.** Do this practice only after you have spent some time in Marsh Grass.

1. Supporting yourself on a noodle, rest passively until your body is warmed and comfortable. Spend at least ten to fifteen minutes. Stabilize yourself by resting your hands on a second noodle, held parallel in front of you, if you like. Review all your muscles to make sure they are relaxed.
2. Visualize your hips swaying about half an inch to the right, but don't do anything. Listen for the message from your back. Wait for permission.
3. If your back invites you, very tentatively, gingerly, allow your hips to sway once, imperceptively, to the right. Induce the movement with your arms and legs, being careful to involve no back muscles.
4. Let your body settle back to neutral. Rest. Review all of your muscles to make sure they are still relaxed.
5. If there were no adverse effects, repeat steps 2 through 4 after a while.
6. Try swaying to the left side. You may find you can sway one way and not the other. It depends on where your spasm has you locked up.

• **Inducing the Natural Curve.** When the lower back is in spasm, the natural curve, or lordosis, can be lost. The lower back becomes flat, or even curved toward the front.

1. Supporting yourself on a noodle, rest passively until your body is warmed and comfortable. Spend at least ten to fifteen minutes. Stabilize yourself by resting your hands on a second noodle, held parallel in front of you, if you like. Review all your muscles to make sure they are relaxed.
2. Visualize your back arching almost imperceptibly, but don't do anything.
3. Listen to your back to see if it grants permission for a little movement. If you get the go-ahead, very tentatively, gingerly, invite your back to return imperceptibly to its natural curve. Imagine that it might arch—just enough to measure—in response to slight movement of your legs and arms. Do not let your back muscles participate.
4. Rest. Review all your muscles. Be sure they are still relaxed.
5. If there were no adverse effects, repeat steps 2 through 4 after a while.

• **Swaying Front to Back.**
1. Supporting yourself on a noodle, rest passively until your body is warmed and comfortable. Spend at least ten to fifteen minutes. Stabilize yourself by resting your hands on a second noodle, held parallel in front of you, if you like. Review all your muscles to make sure they are relaxed.
2. If your back grants permission, invite it, very tentatively, gingerly to curve forward in response to slight movement of your arms and legs. Do not let your back muscles participate.
3. Let your body settle back to neutral. Rest. Review all of your muscles to make sure they are still relaxed.
4. Let your back arch ever so slightly in response to slight movement of your arms and legs. Do not let your back muscles participate.
5. Let your body settle back to neutral. Rest. Review all of your muscles to make sure they are still relaxed.
6. If there were no adverse effects, alternate swaying forward and back. As your back heals, it will let you know how much to increase this motion.

• **Good Neighbors.** If your back problem is sufficiently isolated, you can protect it while practicing very gentle stretches in other parts of your body. I am sometimes able to loosen my upper back and shoulders considerably without involving my lower back. For some reason, relaxing and loosening other muscle groups seems to soothe my lower back. I stress that I am very cautious.

Foot and ankle stretches, for example, could be Good Neighbors. So could Complementary Practices, which are discussed briefly in Part Six.

During the healing period after the spasm has abated, while your muscles are stiff and sore, continue to give yourself plenty of time for passive flotation in warm. Start with **Marsh Grass** and move to gentle forward and backward stretches and side stretches, very gradually intensifying them. Then move gradually into other back stretches.

After the back episode is over, and you are getting back to regular activity, consider practicing postures and stretches that increase the flexibility of your hips as well as your back. Flexibility in the hips is crucial to minimizing strain in the back.

Also consider practicing stretches that focus on your shoulders, upper back and neck. All of the muscles in your body are interactive. Others have worked doubly hard while your back muscles were out of commission.

Finally, identify any posture problems so that you can start to correct them as soon as your back tells you you are able.

DIARY OF WATERYOGA PRACTICE
BACK SPASMS; COMPLEMENTARY PRACTICES

PRACTICE DATE										
Lengthening the Spine										
Marsh Grass										
Swaying to the Side										
Inducing the Natural Curve										
Swaying Front to Back										
Good Neighbors										
Progr. Muscle Relax'n Tech										
Deep Breathing										
Breathing Without Breathing										
Paradoxical Breathing										
Hissing										
Head and Face Massage										
Trapezius Massage										
Abdominal Massage										
Kidney Massage										
Knee Massage										
Meditation										
Body Messages										
Imaging, Visualization										

Affirmations

Carry-Over to Everyday Life

COMMENTS AND SELF-ASSESSMENT

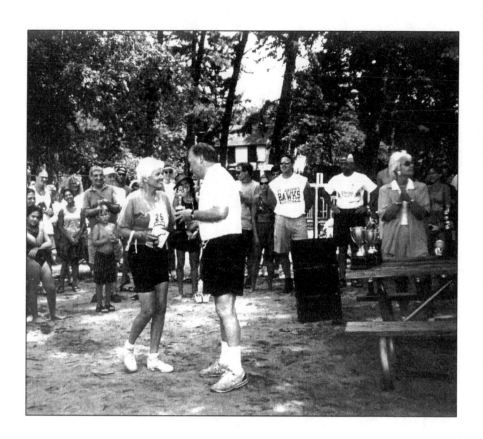

Photograph 10. Jill after her first triathlon. Jill says:

As my back improved with WaterYoga practice, so did my endurance. As my flexibility increased I could ride my bicycle faster, and I could walk naturally again. I decided to celebrate this vast improvement by trying to do a triathlon. But I had not been able to run in all the twenty years that triathlons have been popular.

Swimming and cycling went smoothly. After that I walked the running segment. At sixty-five years old, I did my very first triathlon! Every time I look at this picture, I think again how grateful I am to WaterYoga. It has given me back my life. I will be pleased if WaterYoga helps you too.

PART SIX:

COMPLEMENTARY PRACTICES

The practices described here cannot be treated thoroughly. For more depth, read about them in books and articles in which they are the primary subject.

1. BODY AWARENESS IN EVERYDAY LIFE

Your body will remember the improved posture that you were able to adopt in WaterYoga. Try to retain that posture as you leave the pool. Take your mental image of proper body alignment with you. Try to reflect it in your everyday posture. Your body will imprint itself with good posture while you are in the water and try to approximate it when out of the water.

Your body will also remember the mental equilibrium and spiritual balance that may come with WaterYoga. Remind yourself to take them with you, too, into the rest of life.

What you learn in the water will serve you well later as you sit and stand at your activities in daily life, even while driving your car or sitting in a chair reading. Try Mountain while you are waiting in line at the grocery store. Try Stress Management when the line doesn't move and you are late for an appointment.

2. STRESS MANAGEMENT

Mental stress increases muscle tension, physically stressing them and making them more vulnerable to strain and injury. Stress is increasingly linked to physical disease, especially heart disease and high blood pressure. Oppositely, it has also been shown that positive emotions augment the body's natural defense system, tending to reduce stress, pain and disease.

Mary Pullig Schatz, M.D., author of BACK CARE BASICS, differentiates the bodily stress called the "flight-or-fight" response to *external* threat from the relaxing physical response to messages of *internal* safety and security. It would not be surprising to conclude that the body's response to safety and security is to relax muscle tension, reduce blood pressure, calm nerves, decrease anxiety, and even to heal.

WaterYoga itself is conducive to relaxing your muscles. As an added benefit of physical relaxation comes mental and emotional relaxation. That is a giant step toward stress management.

Listen to your muscles' signals of stress. Relax them by consciously tensing, then relaxing them. Relaxing your face may seem minor, but your face houses your outward expression of stress. Assuming a consciously relaxed countenance tends to reduce stress around you, and it also tends to reduce the stress in your own mind and in the rest of your body. You only need to look at your furrowed brow or turned-down mouth in the mirror to see that this is so.

Become aware of the muscles in which you habitually "hold" your tension or stress. After observing your body carefully, you may be able to locate your body's particular tension-culprits. You may not have been aware of their hiding place. Learn to relax the tension-culprits.

One effective tension reducer is simply breathing fully. Observe the quieting effect of taking long, deep breaths. This is pleasant to do in a warm pool, but it can be done anywhere, even when traffic is at a stand-still on the expressway. You can even consciously breathe out the emotion that has made you tense.

Breathe quietly because audible breathing triggers the flight or fight response in the brain. Maintain the erect, open posture that tells others, and therefore tells you, too, that you are relaxed and serene.

• **Progressive Muscle Relaxation Technique.** Relaxation can be interspersed with postures and stretches, or as preparation for them, or at the end of a practice as a "warm-down." This is a popular and effective relaxation technique. You can practice it most easily in Mountain or Supported Zen. In very shallow water you can combine it with the Feldenkrais Relaxation Technique, which is described on page 138.
1. Clench your right hand into a fist. Hold it as hard as you can for twenty or thirty seconds.
2. Relax your right hand.
3. Repeat with your left hand.
4. Tense the muscles of your right arm. Hold for twenty or thirty seconds.
5. Relax, and repeat with your left arm and hand.
6. Follow the same pattern as you progressively tense and relax your feet and legs, buttocks, abdomen, chest, shoulders, neck, and finally your face and head.

3. BREATHING

Good posture improves breathing. Good breathing improves posture. Moshe Feldenkrais argues for this interdependence in AWARENESS THROUGH MOVEMENT on the grounds that the muscles that control the spine also control breathing.

Breathing is effective only when the thorax hangs in proper postural balance with the spine, sternum and head. The ribs are the frame of the thorax and they contain the lungs. They are mobile at both spine and sternum to allow full downward movement of the diaphragm. In effective breathing, many other muscles are also brought into play.

Effective breathing increases intake of oxygen and therefore provides greater energy. It also has psychological benefits, according to many observers. It can contribute to reduction of panic-induced hyperventilation. Its calming effect enhances emotional stability and self-control, not only inwardly, but also in outward image. It reflects in good posture, which in turn creates an air of attractiveness and confidence.

High, shallow breathing is bad technique. If you have had a panic attack, or felt such compelling emotion that you could not catch your breath, you know what the extreme of this kind of breathing feels like. Concentration of inhalation in the high chest requires a lot of work for not much result. Tense shoulders hold the ribs tight and too wide. Tension extends to the neck and jaw. Downward movement of the diaphragm is restricted. This means that lengthening of the rib cage is also restricted. In addition, high, shallow breathing can interfere with the upper circulatory structures, including the heart.

Deep breathing is good technique. In deep breathing, the diaphragm moves down maximally. This induces depth of chest from top to bottom and from front to back, not from side to side. This tends to lower the body's center of gravity. (You probably won't be able to feel this in the weightlessness of water.) It decreases pressure on the heart, circulatory systems and upper digestive tract in the thorax.

Breathing is normally automatic, meaning that you are not aware of it, even though it may shift radically as your need for oxygen changes, but at the instant you become conscious of your breathing it becomes more controllable. This gives you the capability to appear and act calm even in the face of extraordinary physical or mental demand. It also means that you can educate your body to breathe properly when breathing automatically.

The diaphragm is the key to breathing. Like the psoas muscle, the diaphragm is a major, but often anonymous character in the great body drama. We don't see it bulging right under the skin, we can seldom palpate it. We only know it by its unceasing work on our behalf. The diaphragm is a muscular partition between the thoracic cage and the abdominal cavity. It is attached to the lower ribs and to the third and fourth lumbar vertebrae. In breathing, it goes up and down like a piston in a cylinder. It contracts on the downward stroke, and relaxes on the upward stroke. Movement is only a little more than half an inch, even in deep breathing, but you may sense it as much more. Contraction and relaxation of the diaphragm and the abdominal muscles is reciprocal as inhalation and exhalation alternate.

Inhalation is the exertion phase of normal breathing. Its pur pose is to increase the volume of the chest cavity to accept air.

Volume in the chest, as in any other physical structure, has three dimensions: height, width and depth. The chest can enlarge to the front, to the back and to the sides. It cannot expand upward to any helpful extent because at the upper level the lungs are narrow and contained in a rather rigid rib structure. The lowest two ribs, the floating ribs, are not connected to the sternum, and are thus quite movable. They provide most of the volume of inhalation.

When the diaphragm contracts on inhalation, it is drawn down toward its attachment at the lumbar vertebrae, which reduces the curvature of the spine. The abdomen softens and bulges outward to contain the viscera that the diaphragm has pushed ahead of itself. At the same time, the sternum moves forward and upward, bringing with it the forward ends of the connected ribs. The spine moves back to balance the frontal expansion. Sideways expansion is slight, to avoid interference from the arms. Expansion at the upper rib level is also slight, due to the skeletal limitation. The shoulder muscles are only minimally involved in normal breathing

Exhalation is the resting phase of normal breathing. The muscles that caused inhalation relax. This diminishes the volume of the chest cavity, which compresses the lungs, expelling air. The diaphragm rises into the chest. At the same time the abdominal muscles activate.

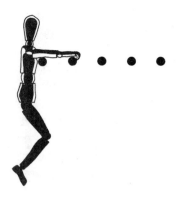

BREATHING TECHNIQUES

You can experiment with the following conscious breathing techniques without any risk of forgetting how to breathe automatically.

• **Deep Breathing.** Start in Mountain.
1. Put one hand on your sternum and the other on your spine at the level of your sternum.
2. Inhale. Identify the muscular activity. Notice the increase in volume of your chest cavity. Pull the top of the sternum toward your head, and out away from your spine. Feel your hands move apart. Let your abdomen expand as your diaphragm descends. Let the bottom of your rib cage expand freely. Do not involve your shoulder girdle.
3. Exhale. This is the rest phase of breathing. Your diaphragm relaxes. Your ribs and sternum lower by their own weight. As a result the lungs are compressed in the decreased volume of the chest cavity. Lengthen your rib muscles and the extensor muscles of your back to keep your rib cage narrow and long. Do not reduce the volume of your chest cavity by leaving your rib cage wide and reducing the length of your spine, which would compress your vertebrae.
4. Repeat, breathing slowly and deeply.
5. Move your hands to the sides of your lower ribs, and breathing slowly and deeply, notice their action.
6. Move your hands as high as you can to the sides of your ribs, and breathing slowly and deeply, notice their action at that level.
7. Move your hands to your back, at the floating ribs, and breathing slowly and deeply, notice their action at that level.
8. Move your hands to your abdomen and solar plexus, or "breadbasket," and breathing slowly and deeply, notice their action.

• **Breathing Without Breathing.** You have to be able to hold
your breath to do this variation on deep breathing. It is a
Feldenkrais exercise designed to increase your awareness of
your body's movements in breathing. Start in Mountain.
1. Go through the physical movements of deep breathing while
   holding your breath. Become aware of the movement of your
   ribs, sternum, abdomen and diaphragm.
2. Forcefully push your abdomen out as your diaphragm
   descends; push your sternum up and out as your diaphragm
   ascends. Visualize your diaphragm pushing the contents of
   your torso alternately into the upper and lower parts of an
   hourglass. But don't overdo. This breathing pattern requires
   exertion.
3. Breathe normally, incorporating the movements of 1 and 2.

• **Paradoxical Breathing.** Feldenkrais describes as "paradoxical" this breathing technique by which the diaphragm moves up
instead of down while the lungs fill. In the Orient, this form of
breathing is thought to improve posture. Paradoxical breathing
is what gives the lion his roar.

Increased exchange of gases in the deep body tissues is also
thought by some to occur during paradoxical breathing, as a
result of increased pressure on the abdomen during exhalation.
Ascension of the diaphragm during inhalation strengthens the
frontal abdominal muscles. When they are strong, the spinal
extensors are freed to support the thoracic vertebrae and
sacrum and help to lengthen the chest cavity.
1. Inhale, slowly expanding the chest using the muscles of the
   rib cage. Tighten the abdomen so that the viscerae force the
   diaphragm up. Expansion should be to the front and back,
   and should not involve the upper rib cage.
2. Exhale, slowly contracting the rib cage and driving the
   diaphragm down into the abdomen. Exhale completely, feeling the pressure as far down as the floor of the abdominal
   cavity.
3. Repeat several times with a long rhythm, but don't overdo.
   This breathing pattern requires exertion.

• **Hissing.** I associate hissing, which Mabel E. Todd describes in her book THINKING BODY with the Paradoxical Breathing that Feldenkrais describes in AWARENESS THROUGH MOVE-MENT.

1. Inhale as in Paradoxical Breathing.
2. Exhale while hissing like a snake, driving your diaphragm deep into your abdomen. Feel its impact all the way down to your rectum. Hissing helps the psoas muscles, spinal extensors and rib muscles to deepen and narrow the rib cage. Sense the ribs moving back and down. The psoas is a very big player here.
3. Breathe several times this way with a long rhythm. Image your spine lengthening, as a consequence of your body narrowing. Don't overdo. This breathing pattern requires exertion.
4. Next, on a few exhalations, make a low guttural sound at the back of your throat instead of hissing.
5. Breathe several times this way with a long rhythm, but don't overdo this either.

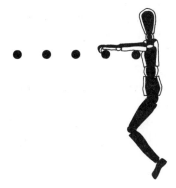

4. MASSAGE

More and more people are realizing that there is just nothing more relaxing than a good massage. Therapists are developing forms of massage for use in the water. The one I have been told about is called Watsu, for which therapists are now being specially trained.

What I offer in this section is a few examples of self-massage, which I sometimes incorporate in my WaterYoga practice when I have the luxury of a lot of time in the warm pool. You can also do these massage techniques in your tub or shower, or anywhere you can submerge for long enough to warm your hands and body.

• **Head and Face Massage.** Stand in Mountain. The benefit will be greater if you keep your eyes closed. Don't worry if you drift off balance. Just stand up again.
1. Gently smoothe your face—from your nose outward to your ears. Very gently rub the area under the eyes. Never rub the eyes themselves. Squint and blink your eyes.
2. Cover your eyes for a minute with your hands. Roll them, lids closed, clockwise, then counterclockwise. (Some eastern practitioners advocate breathing in while rolling from nine o'clock to three o'clock and breathing out from three o'clock to nine o'clock. This is said to benefit the inner organs as well as the eyes.)
3 Gently rub your temples in a circular motion; smoothe your chin line up to the ears, smoothe your forehead toward your hairline.
4. Cup your right hand over your right ear with just enough pressure that your head must resist. Hold. Repeat, cupping your left ear with your left hand.
5. Gently massage the back of your neck at the base of your skull.
6. Run your tongue around the outside of your teeth several times, clockwise and counterclockwise. Then twist your tongue clockwise and counterclockwise.

• **Trapezius Massage**.

1. Massage your left upper trapezius muscle (which runs roughly from the top of the left shoulder joint to the neck) with the right hand, keeping your left shoulder down and relaxed. For a more vigorous massage, continue to massage as you move your left shoulder in big circles, forward and backward.
2. Repeat, massaging the right trapezius muscle with the left hand.

• **Abdominal Massage.** The abdomen is said to be the source of the vital energy called Ch'i. But caution: if you have been diagnosed with an aortal aneurism, or if your physician believes that your risk of one is high, do not massage the abdomen.

1. Gently rub your abdomen in a circular motion with your hands. This stimulates the abdominal muscles and intestinal circulation.
2. Gently place both palms against your middle abdomen and breathe into their pressure. This is said to relieve pains of constipation and menstruation.

• **Kidney Massage**.

1. Vigorously rub the palms of your hands on your back, just above the waist.

• **Knee Massage**.

1. Lean against a wall, or sit in shallow water (perhaps on the steps into a thermal pool).
2. Rub each thigh and knee in a circular motion from inside to outside.

5. MEDITATION

WaterYoga, like traditional forms of yoga, can include a med-itational component. Studies indicate that meditation can decrease metabolism, lower blood pressure, slow down some brain waves, slow down respiration and slow down pulse.

The extent to which you introduce meditation into your WaterYoga practice is entirely your own preference. Sometimes I meditate and sometimes I don't (as when there are interesting people to talk to in the pool).

Meditation facilitates your ability to focus your mind on your postures and stretches, and even on the sensations of your skin and muscle. This is called kinesthesia. To meditate, simply focus your mind on the posture or stretch in which you are engaged. Be entirely mindful of it. If your thoughts wander, simply return them. That is meditation in its simplest form.

Many meditation systems are built around the repetition of a word, sound or mantra. It may be repeated silently or aloud.

Meditation may also be as simple as observing your breath-ing—inhaling and exhaling. Breathe regularly in and out, but not so roughly as to be heard. Do not hold your breath. Breathe through your nose, naturally, slowly, inaudibly, moderately deeply. Or you may inhale through your nose, and exhale through your mouth. Experience the feelings in your chest and abdomen as air goes in and out. Concentrate on the inner ener-gy in your abdomen as it receives oxygen. Diminish your thoughts by turning inward to your breathing, in and out, in and out.

You may close your eyes, or if you keep your eyes open, keep your focus "softened" and slightly downward, helping you to become "inward-centered." Consciously keep your jaw relaxed. Gritting your teeth is a sure sign of tension.

Concentrate your mind two inches below your navel. Be in no hurry, and do not expect any results at all. Empty your mind. Maintain a quiet centering within yourself. Images will come into your mind—it's never truly "empty." Don't try to keep them out, but just allow them to go away. Count your breaths if that helps to clear the images from your mind.

Your mind has room only for what is in the here and now. Doing your postures and stretches is all there is. "Progress," "success," "failure," "purpose," "effort" are outside of the here and now. Your mind, like your body, becomes quiet and stable, concentrating, without effort, on what you are doing here, in this moment.

Zen meditation is an ancient and simple way to meditate. It is easily transferred to the water, and therefore very beneficial to WaterYoga. It can be said to be only this: when you do something, do it with your whole mind and body. Leave everything else outside. Enter the reality of the present moment, leaving behind both past and future.

There is no need to understand Zen intellectually, no need to concentrate on any particular state of mind. Concentration itself is tiring, if you concentrate on anything specific. So concentrate on nothing except your breathing. But make no effort to concentrate. Here is the essence of Zen in breathing: if you keep your mind on your breathing, you will become unaware of your breathing. Don't worry if this instruction seems contradictory. In Zen, the two sides of a contradiction are but the two sides of a single coin.

Although it may be self-defeating to try for them, some people may, in the course of the physical practice of meditation, perceive spiritual and mental benefits.

6. BODY-MESSAGES

Your thoughts and feelings are reflected in your posture. You "tell" about your mental and emotional state to others by the way you move and stand. This has been called "body language." Conversely, it can also be said that your movements and posture influence your own thoughts and feelings. If this is so, your physical posture affects your fundamental personality! Be aware that good thoughts and good attitudes affect your body for the better. An erect head, relaxed shoulders, and calm breathing reveal energy and confidence.

Good body alignment, which is another way of saying good posture, sends a positive message of attitude to your own mind. Consider the figure of speech "a mental slump." A forward body slump reflects depression. Does it also *intensify* depression? I think so. Within the oneness of your body and mind/spirit, there is reciprocity between your physical posture and your mental attitude. Barbara Hoberman Levine says it well in her book, YOUR BODY BELIEVES EVERY WORD YOU SAY.

Since correct posture is of central interest in the practice of WaterYoga, the language of the basic posture in WaterYoga (as well as in traditional forms of yoga) asks us to lift our sternum, lift our head, lift each vertebra for physical separation. In the oneness of yoga, the lifting of the body asks us to lift the spirit and mind as well. Consider that a blue mood is over when it "lifts."

Here's another mind-body connection: a smile (physical action) brightens mood (emotional state). Make a smile part of your WaterYoga. It is almost impossible to smile and slump at the same time. Extend the smile to your attitudes and thoughts. Extend it to your neighbors. As little children learn to sing:

"If you're happy and you know it
Then your face will surely show it."

7. IMAGING; VISUALIZATION

Body-messages are the external expression of "imaging" or visualization. I use these two terms interchangeably. Visualization can create in your mind an image of the healing of any sick part of your body.

Visualize your posture improving, your muscles relaxing, your spine lengthening as the discs take in nourishment. Visualize your joints opening up.

Form an image of the blocked-up tension in your body. Then visualize it actually running out of your jaw, or out of your fingers and your toes, washing away from you in the warm water.

Visualize your arthritis (or posture or circulation) improving as you practice WaterYoga. Visualize yourself with perfect posture, perfect alignment, flexibility, strength, and confidence. But be aware that your internal sensory imaging and visualization may not be accurate. This is why it is important to stay in touch with your health care professional for periodic check-ups.

Bruce Kodish, one of the many kind reviewers of this manuscript, and a teacher of the Alexander Technique, points out that imaging can also be done as an opposite: "becoming aware of and letting go of what you are doing 'wrong' might help the 'right' thing to do itself."

8. AFFIRMATIONS

Affirmations are simply instructions to your own mind, spirit and body. You can say them aloud, or think them to yourself. Try repeating affirmations during postures and stretches such as:

"my back is open now so the nerve isn't so pinched.
I feel the space open up,"

or,

"I am relaxing. . .relaxing. . .relaxing. . . ."

Your affirmation may influence the reality. Affirmations can be combined with imaging, or with meditation, as well as with your postures and stretches.

Barbara Hoberman Levine, in YOUR BODY BELIEVES EVERY WORD YOU SAY, agrees with Frank Sinatra's song that we must accentuate health-affirming thoughts and eliminate unhealthy ones. Make this especially true as you practice WaterYoga.

PART SEVEN

GLOSSARY AND ADDITIONAL INFORMATION

I have tried to include material here that I think will be helpful to you in thinking about WaterYoga. Some parts of it may be more than you would ever want to know; other parts may be a dull rehash of what you already know. I put in the long section on Baths and Spas over the objection of almost all of the people who read this manuscript, for the simple reason that I found it fascinating.

I am sure that this Glossary is not all-inclusive. Go to the Resources section for more depth and detail in your study.

Acupressure. Acupressure is an adaptation of acupuncture (which see). Its principle is the same, but its technique is pressure on the surface of the skin by a practitioner. If you are morbidly afraid of needles, you may find acupressure helpful. Acupressure can also be taught for self treatment.

Acupuncture. Acupuncture is an ancient oriental procedure for treatment and prevention of various medical conditions, and for promotion of well-being. For example, it addresses stress, headache, some neuralgias, neck pain, lower back pain, sciatica, arthritis, frozen shoulder, tendonitis, sinusitis, sore throat, bronchitis, cough, asthma, digestive disorders, urinary, menstrual and reproductive complaints, and even obesity, addictions and insomnia. Its principle is stimulation and balancing of energy flow throughout the body. Its technique is insertion of hair-thin sterile needles into appropriate "points" along the "meridians" of flow of Ch'i (which see).An interesting aspect of acupuncture for the skeptical westerner is that there is no need to believe that acupuncture will work.

Alexander Technique. The Alexander Technique was developed by an Australian, F. Matthias Alexander, in the late nineteenth century. He held his first training class in 1933 and continued to teach until he died at the age of 86.

The Alexander Technique is an effortless mind-body experience that claims to unlock the flow of physical, mental and spritual energy, improve the sense of well-being, increase grace, flexibility and ease, and lessen fatigue. This occurs in the interaction of feeling, thinking and physical reactions in the unified being. Observable physical results are improved alignment and posture. As the back lengthens and widens, muscles that are accustomed to being tense and tight are retaught to let go and become free.

The essence of the Alexander Technique is the mind's instruction to the body: "Let the neck be free to let the head go forward and up, to let the back lengthen and widen." If the head cannot go forward and up, the spine cannot lengthen.

The Alexander Technique is not a cure or a treatment, but a series of lessons in which you learn how to move in all activities, simple and complex; to use your body (actually your self, which includes your mind) well. The process involves relearning basic movements: sitting, standing, walking, bending, reaching, lifting, and even lying down. It involves understanding that what you *sense* you are doing is not necessarily what you *are* doing. The Alexander Technique is applicable to all the phases of life: emotional and mental as well as postural.

Allopathic Medicine. *Allo* is a Greek word meaning "other" or differing from the normal or usual. Allopathic medicine uses substitutive therapy. A disease is treated by producing a morbid reaction of another kind or in another part. It is a healing practice that generally treats symptoms instead of cause.

Arthritis. Most inflammatory diseases of the joints are lumped under the general heading of arthritis. They can exhibit quite different symptoms, and therefore require quite different treatment and care.

Ayurvedic Medicine. Ayurveda means "science of life." It is the health care system of Hinduism in India, said to be 5,000 years old, or perhaps almost 10,000. Its themes are holism, prevention, and harmony with all living forms. It addresses the essential nature and meaning of life because its practitioners believe that divine life force and creative intelligence are present to form each individual.

Baths and Spas. Warm water has a curative and salutary history as long as that of yoga, but unfortunately, its history has gotten lost along with the archaic use of the word "bath." I am indebted to the Encyclopedia Brittanica, 11th edition, 1910, for most of this information.

In the western world, salutary and healing effects of warm water have been known since the golden age of the Greeks, who built pools to contain the water of thermal springs. For example, Thermopylae (which means "hot gate") is chiefly known for the Spartans' defense of it against the Persian army of Xerxes, but its name tells us that it was known before that for its hot springs. The Greek writer, Homer, noted that warm baths were used after fatigue or exercise. Vestiges of Greek construction can be seen even today, as in a thermal spring in Provence, near the Mediterranean coast of France.

"Taking the baths" was popular as recently as 1910, and was said to "produce good effects for rheumatism." Taking the baths was also said to relieve sciatica, gout, paralysis, neuralgia, internal complaints such as kidney stones and uric acid, sciatica, diseases of the liver, and "skin affections [sic].

In order to understand the concept of taking the baths, you must first understand the original English meaning of the word "bath." According to the Encyclopedia Britannica edition of 1910, "a bath is the immersion of the body in a medium different from the ordinary one of atmospheric air, which medium is usually common water in some form." Thus, a "bath" includes all forms of application of water, vapor, sand, chemicals, even electricity, to the body.

In the nineteenth century "bathing" at the shore became popular. Swimming as we know it was just one way to take a bath at the shore. So the first swimming pools were called "swimming baths." We still sun-bathe and take a mud-bath.

Without this bit of etymology, it is hard to appreciate the salutary value of "taking a bath." It perhaps even got mixed up with cleansing as curative. But in long past centuries, baths were so important that wherever the Romans extended their Empire, they built baths. Baths that were fed by naturally hot springs were called *"thermae"* (hot). By extension, baths that were heated by furnaces came also to be called thermae. [The Roman baths whose waters were supplied by aqueducts or rivers were called *"piscinae"* (for fish). In French today, a swimming pool is a *"piscine."*]

Many Roman thermae contained swimming baths, warm baths, hot air baths and vapor baths. The elaborate engineering of their furnaces tells us how greatly the Romans valued the salutary effect of warm water. They often included gymnasia, social rooms and even libraries. The elegance of their architecture and decoration attests to the significance of leisure and pleasure that accompanied the bath. The sumptuous Baths of Caracala, including furnaces and other rooms, were a quarter of a mile square and contained "seats" for 1600 bathers. The bathing process came no closer to washing than "water being poured . . . over [the] head, . . .[the skin] next to be scraped with the *strigil* . . . ." (a blunt, rather knife-like instrument with a curved blade, used to remove sweat and dirt during a hot bath.) The modern validity of this 2000 year old practice is beautifully demonstrated by the present popularity of astringents in skin care. " Astringent" is derived from the present participle of the related latin verb *astringere.*

"Bath" is derived from an ancient European word most akin to "bake." This is evidence that the property of warmth was central to early use of warm springs as baths. Bath, in England, can be traced to Roman remains called *Aqua Sulis* (Water of Minerva) in the province of Britannia. It was named in honor of a goddess in gratitude for the benefits and pleasures of the waters. Its temperature ranged from 117 to 120 degrees F.

A little-known fact confirms the importance of the concept of Bath to English history: no heir can ascend the throne of Great Britain without having first been awarded the Order of the Bath in a grand fur- and sword-draped ceremony in Westminster Abbey.

France (Gaul) has three towns named *"Agua"* by the Romans for their warm healing springs. Agua was corrupted to the modern "Aix" (-en-Provence, -la-Chappelle, and -les-Bains). *"Bains"* means baths in French.

With the decadence of Roman society and the rise of early Christian asceticism, "bathing" fell into disfavor. Turkey, Egypt and even Russia, however, less influenced by Christian Rome, continued the use of thermal baths, building extensive facilities in their own lavish architectural styles. Some people still refer to "Turkish Baths."

In the United States, two notable towns are called Hot Springs. One is in Bath (!) County, Virginia (temperatures as high as 106 degrees F.), and the other is in Arkansas (temperature ranging from 95 - 147 degrees F.). In New York State, there is Saratoga Springs. In Georgia, Warm Springs became prominent when President Franklin Roosevelt found relief from the pain of polio (then called infantile paralysis) in its waters. There are also warm springs in California, Colorado, West Virginia, Florida and Idaho. I am sure I have left some out.

In German, *bad* means "bath," or "watering place." Baden was the most elegant "watering place" in Austria, having thirteen naturally warm baths, which gave the town its name. Baden dates to the Roman era, when it was called *Thermae Pannonicae* (Pannonia was a Roman colony located south of the Danube River). To distinguish itself from Austria's Baden, a warm spring in the Black Forest of Germany called itself

Baden-_Baden._ It has twenty-two hot springs, which are "accounted the most elegant in Europe."

The modern word "spa" means a fashionable resort with mineral springs. It is derived from the name of a town in Belgium, where mineral springs were discovered in 1326. All later-named spas are reputed to be named for Spa. In Spa and many other places as far flung as Uruguay, Buda-Pest and Wales, bathing buildings are great monuments to the salutary effects of warm water.

Modern public water systems do not contain the minerals that are found in the water of the old spas and baths. These minerals include sulfur, calcium, sodium sulfates, and sodium and magnesium chlorides. It has never been determined that they are actually helpful. Research should be done in this area.

Breathing. Two lungs are located in the human thorax. They are alternately filled (inhalation) so that the body may harvest oxygen for fuel, and emptied (exhalation) so that the body can discard carbon dioxide. The lungs themselves have no muscles, but are filled and emptied by surrounding bones and muscles. The surrounding bones are the ribs, sternum, and spine. The muscles that control those bones are the muscles of the upper chest, back of the neck, and ribs; and the major unnoticed player, the diaphragm. Because all the muscle groups of the body work together, the muscles of the trunk, arms, legs, back, pelvis and abdomen are also involved in breathing.

Lung capacity is more than a gallon of air (visualize a gallon jug of milk). But when the body is not taxed, each inhaled breath is probably not more than a pint (visualize a pint of cream). The lungs cannot ever be completely emptied. There is always a residual pint or so of air in them.

Breathing patterns change automatically to meet the physical demands of strenuous exertion such as sex, pain, childbirth, sports, etc. They also change automatically to meet emotional demands such as fear, doubt, mental effort, grief, concentration. As to how we breathe, we pant, gasp, sigh, yawn, sniff, sneeze, snort, groan, hyperventilate, hiccup. The variations are endless. We even stop breathing entirely. But the automatic breathing stimulus saves us from suffocating. It is virtually impossible to hold your breath until you suffocate.

Buoyancy. See Physics.

Chest. See Thorax.

Ch'i. There is no English word that exactly corresponds to the word "Ch'i." Many health care systems in the Eastern traditions believe that keeping the body flexible and relaxed aids in the circulation of the vital, life energy ("Ch'i"), which leads to greater health and tends to prevent illness and the incapacities of old age. These systems believe that Ch'i sustains, nourishes and balances all the organs in the body. Ch'i is known in many cultures, including the African and the American Indian. Hindu Yogis call it Prana. Japanese call it Ki. Ch'i also corresponds to the Hebrew word *ruach.*

Ch'i circulates through well-defined "meridians," or channels in the body. Although no physical presentation of Ch'i has yet been conclusively discovered, recent medical evidence supports the notion that it does somehow "exist."

Ch'i is the starting point for application of Chinese medicine. A major principle of acupuncture is the balancing of Ch'i through insertion of slender needles in acupuncture points along these meridians.

Focusing on breathing turns the mind away from external stimuli, and centers the mind/spirit in the chest and especially in the abdomen, which is considered to be the source of Ch'i.

Chiropractic. Chiropractic is a strongly manipulative treatment of the spine, directed to improved alignment of vertebrae or other bones. It is based on the theory that the well-being of the body is dependent on the condition of the spine, and that good alignment of the back and the spine is necessary to good body function, to prevention of backaches, slipped discs, muscle spasm and many other ailments that may not appear to be directly related to the spine and back.

Disc. See Spine.

Feldenkrais Method. Dr. Moshe Feldenkrais (1904-1984) developed two body movement and posture systems called Awareness Through Movement and Functional Integration in the late 1940s. A physicist and judo expert, he took a psychophysical approach (body and mind) in creating an ingenious variety of rolling, turning, bending and rocking exercises, combined with deep breathing. These exercises are designed to release and amend fixed body habits. The Feldenkrais Method is said to increase ease and range of motion, improve flexibility and coordination, and develop the innate capacity for graceful, efficient movement.

Feldenkrais had taken Alexander lessons, and his approach is consistent with the Alexander Technique, but he also concentrated on strengthening the back muscles, on the theory that a strong back is necessary for efficient body usage.

Feldenkrais work consists of teaching and reeducation rather than treatment, and involves mind and body in both method and results. Movements range from tiny movements to large acrobatic movements: sometimes there is no movement and only the imagination is used to bring changes into the body. The movements are performed without strain, without trying to reach a goal, and some exercises seem to have no connection with the original body movement. There is constant awareness of *how* one is moving and where change is taking place. "Do less than what you can do" is a common Feldenkrais instruction.

Gravity. See Physics; see Posture and Human Physics.

Hip Joint. The hip joint has two functions. It is both a weight-bearing structure and a movable joint. Distribution of the load of upper-body weight from the pelvis occurs at the two hip joints. It is also a hinge joint, enabling the body to sit, bend, and walk or run. Both of these rather inconsistent structural functions are vital to human posture and motion.

Because the pelvis slopes forward and the pelvic slope continues through the necks of the femurs, or thigh bones, weight transfers through the hip joints down the thighs on a plane about 2 1/2 inches in front of the lumbosacral joint. In the upright position, the entire weight of the body above it sits on the heads of the femurs. The femur, which is the body's longest bone, is controlled and moved by muscles attached far up the trunk and along the spine. A strong hip joint is, therefore, vital to posture and movement.

Mobility in the hip joints is also vital because it allows the body to bend without straining the back. Lack of mobility in the hip necessitates compensatory movement in the spine, mainly at the fourth and fifth lumbar vertebrae. See also Pelvis and Pelvic Basin.

Holistic Health Care. Whole treatment; care of the entire patient in all aspects. Holistic health care is based on the theory that body, mind, and spirit all play interlocking roles in health.

Homeopathy. *Homeo* is from a Greek word meaning "like, or similar," and *pathy* is from a Greek word meaning "illness." Homeopathy is a system of therapy developed by Samuel Hahnemann in which disease is treated by administration of small doses of minerals, herbs and other substances that create the symptoms of the disease itself. Its basic theory is "the law of similars." I liken it to "jump-starting" a car, in that it stimulates the natural defenses of the body to heal itself.

Hydrostatic Pressure. See Physics.

Hydrotherapy. *Hydro* means water, so hydrotherapy is any form of treatment in water. It was first used by Hippocrates in the fourth century B.C. In classical times, medicine was typically practiced in the public baths. (See Baths and Spas.)

Iyengar Yoga. B. K. S. Iyengar is the innovator of a rigorous school of Hatha Yoga. It is based on thorough and intimate knowledge of the body. It makes use of props such as straps, wooden blocks, bolsters, folded blankets, and even chairs. Walls are often "props," too. Emphasis is on the proper postural alignment of the physical body.

Four books by Iyengar illustrate the hundreds of poses that he teaches: LIGHT ON PRANAYAMA, TREE OF YOGA, LIGHT ON YOGA and LIGHT ON THE YOGA SUTRAS OF PATANJALI. These books support Iyengar's teaching that Yoga is also a purificatory process, beyond mere physical care, leading one to the ability "to feel and enjoy heaven on the plane of earth." (quoted from Yoga Journal May/June 1995 p. 65) (And see Yoga.)

Kinesthesia. Kinesthesia is one's sensory awareness of muscles, tendons and joints as they are stimulated by one's body movement and tension. It includes bodily reaction and motor memory.

Ligament. Ligaments, in a simplified definition, are the powerful tissues that connect the bones to each other.

Lung. See Breathing.

Pelvis and Pelvic Basin. The pelvis is a massive cup-shaped ring of bone, with its ligaments, at the lower end of the trunk. It is attached to the spine at the sacrum. Pelvis, which means basin in Latin, is the basin that holds the abdominal and pelvic cavities. Its bones are the pubis in the front; ilium and ischium on the side; and sacrum and coccyx in the back. It hangs as a side load on the compression members at the back of the trunk. It is properly balanced when the spine pulls down and tensile members at the front pull up. The forward slope of the pelvis is not evident on exterior observation of the body, but shows clearly in a side view of the skeleton.

The pelvic area is also the focus for attachments of muscles used for standing, sitting and walking. This means that the pelvic muscles must be large and strong. About thirty-six muscles are attached to the pelvis. They run well up into the trunk and down into the legs. Besides their moving functions, they help to support the body wall. They unite the main body-blocks, joining thorax, trunk, legs, and even the head, with the pelvis.

The pelvic ligaments, particularly those related to the hip joint, also support the spine, reinforcing the attachment of the lumbar spine to the sacrum and the sacrum to the ilia and ischia.

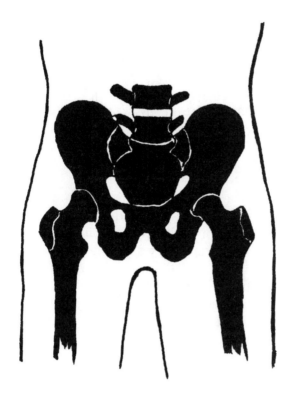

Illustration 72. Pelvis (skeleton)

Physics. Archimedes' Principle states that the weight of a mass is virtually the same as the weight of the mass of water it displaces. In the human body, fat and air or other gases in the tissues and organs are lighter than water. Muscles and bones are heavier than water. Different people are constituted of fat, muscle, bone and gases in different proportions, which is why some people are "sinkers" and others are "floaters."

Water has a specific gravity of 1. It is the benchmark against which all other matter is measured. A heavy metal, like lead, has a specific gravity greater than 1. Lead sinks in water. Cork has a specific gravity less than 1. A cork floats in water. The average human body, with air in the lungs, has a specific gravity of .974, and thus is very slightly lighter than water.

Buoyancy is upward force on a mass immersed in a fluid. Buoyancy acts in the opposite direction from gravity. It assists in any motion toward the surface and resists any downward motion. The buoyancy of your body in water is determined by the weight of the water that the mass of your body displaces.

Hydrostatic pressure is the pressure that the surrounding water exerts equally on every surface of your body while it is immersed in water. This pressure is greater the deeper you are in the water. SCUBA divers experience a demonstrable compression of the body when they dive to fifty or a hundred feet.

Resistance is the opposing force of some other medium or object. Water offers slight and yielding resistance to the movement of a body through it. Strangely, it is resistance to the push of arms and legs against the water that enables a swimmer to move through the water. At the same time, the less resistance the swimmer's body offers, the more efficiently it overcomes resistance to swim faster. This is why swimmers "streamline." Streamlining is related to the axis of gravity and is therefore important to posture.

Still air offers no significant resistance to the body's movement. Wind, however, creates resistance. The prayer of the bicyclist is: "May the wind be ever at your back." Floors and walls, however, create essentially absolute resistance to your push. In isotonic weight training, you strengthen muscles by pushing something heavy against gravity. Weight training is strenuous exercise.

Posture and Human Physics. In the physical universe, gravity is ever-present. Gravity causes downward pressure. Transfer of the weight of any structure is ultimately downward, and causes compression in the structure. "Compression members" carry the force of the weight downward.

Downward pressure on a structure must be equalled by upward thrust, or the structure will collapse to the ground. Tensile members are suspensory parts which pull the weight of the structure to higher points on the compression members, where it is received and transferred to the ground. Look at the nearest suspension bridge, or your back yard swing, to see these principles in action. All of this happens in relation to the gravitational axis of the structure: that is, the straight vertical line on all sides of which the structure's weight is balanced.

In addition to compression and tension, three other forces affect the gravitational axis. They are torsion (twist, as when you look behind you while driving a car), shear (sliding of one part upon another, as when you jut your chin forward) and bending. Every force must be counteracted by an equal force in the opposite direction.

These forces represent the challenge that the laws of physics present to the human body. The challenge is hard to meet for at least two reasons:

(1) The human body is not a unitary compression member, like a telephone pole. If it were, it would be rigid. Movement would be impossible. Contrast the stiffness of a telephone pole with a string of beads. Contrast a praying mantis with a snake. Br'er Snake's spine is strung like beads on a string. You can hold a string of beads upright, but as soon as you drop it it collapses in a heap. The difference between Br'er Snake and a string of beads is that he has muscles. The difference between Br'er Snake and a telephone pole is that he has joints.

(2) Human arms and legs and organs have to be supported on this vertical axis. And they do not sit on top of the compression member, the spine, but are ranged around it. And they move a whole lot.

A structure can support weight in three ways. Weight can sit, hang, or be braced. The human skeleton supports weight in all three ways: the head sits atop the spine in a simple "top-load," the arms hang from the shoulder girdle, and the hipbones (ilia) brace, or take the transverse load from, the sacrum, in what is called a "side-load."

The human body's axis of gravity is the central line, or line of balance when the body mass is stable, down which the load of its weight travels to the ground. It is another law of physics that the nearer to center the weight is maintained, the less energy must be spent to keep it balanced. The anatomical body, too, has a best mechanical position for balance. (See illustrations on pages 21, 22 and 23.) Movement of any one part away from the gravitational axis of the body involves the movement of an equal part in an opposite direction. That's why you have to stick your other arm out when you carry a bucket of water.

The front wall of the trunk is composed mostly of tensile members: muscles, fascia and other soft tissues. Here there is no successive "sitting" of body weights one atop another, from head to pelvis, as there is in the spinal structure in the back. Instead, (a) upward traction of the tensile members balances the compression members of the spine, (b) the pelvis is partly suspended from the thorax by the front-wall abdominal muscles, and (c) the thoracic cage and shoulder girdle are suspended from the head and neck by a system of muscles and tendons. This converts a considerable portion of the trunk weight into a top-load, carried up to the head and back down through the compression members of the spinal column. The upward pull of these tensile members in front and the downward compression forces in the back should be equal.

All muscles that tend to straighten the back have complementary muscles tending to bend it toward the front, as the laws of physics require. Defective posture habits lead to habitually strained muscles and a lack of balance of the bones at the joints. The deep iliopsoas muscles, which attach the legs to the inner sides of the spine, and the strong abdominal muscles, which attach to the pelvic rim and run up in front to the ribs and the breastbone, act together as tensile members to hold the pelvis in the best position to receive the weight passing to it from the sacrum. If they are weak, the muscles at the back of the spine will have to make up their deficit. Their increased tension will tend to lift the load at the sacrum, which will open up the sides of the pelvic arch at the keystone. These muscles are extensors; their function is to pull down and back, not up and forward. If they are forced to do the wrong job, damage may result.

Psoas. The psoas is a major tensile muscle, perhaps the most important of all the muscles in the human's upright posture. *(Psoas* comes from the Greek word for "muscles of the loins." "Lumbar" means loins in Latin.) The psoas muscle is associated with the iliopsoas muscle. On each side of the deep abdominal cavity it follows the frontal side of the lumbar spine up to the twelfth thoracic vertebra, attaches to all the lumbar vertebrae, and descends into the thigh. See page 71 for illustration.

Resistance. See Physics.

Rolfing. Rolfing was developed by Ida Rolf. It is a treatment that consists of intense manipulative body massage. It is also called deep tissue massage. Body posture is changed through severe pressure, and as a result, alignment and movement are generally improved. For most people, it is quite painful. Rolfing works on the connective tissue, which connects muscle to muscle and muscle to bone. According to Rolf, this connective tissue has shortened abnormally when a body has had poor alignment, and must be restored to length and elasticity.

Referred Pain. Pain is said to be "referred" when it is felt in a different location in the body from its source. This is frequently the case in nerve pain.

Sciatica. Sciatica is pain down the haunch and leg that radiates from the sciatic nerve. The sciatic nerve goes out of the spine between the 4th and 5th lumbar vertebrae. When it is pinched or inflamed the pain is generated, often far down the course of the nerve.

Scoliosis. Scoliosis is a sideways curvature of the spine. It is more common in females than in males. It usually causes no discomfort in childhood, but can get worse in adults. Problems most often found in adults with scoliosis are back pain, arthritic changes in the spine, and a tendency for the lateral curves to slowly increase, with consequent loss of height, balance and space within the torso. Scoliosis can be either a C curve, or an S curve. See page 24 for illustration.

Shiatsu. Shiatsu is an oriental discipline of gentle stretching and joint mobilization.

Spa. See Bath.

Shoulders and Shoulder Girdle. The shoulder girdle is a bony, yoke-like arrangement, hung across the top of the thoracic cage (rather like a lamp-shade that attaches at the finial). It consists of two clavicles (Latin: small key) and two scapulae, and lies outside the chest wall. The clavicles are attached to the top of the sternum. The sternum is connected with the spinal column through the ribs. Thus, the shoulder girdle itself does not connect with the bones of the spine except through the clavicles to the sternum to the ribs. See pages 60 and 61 for illustrations.

The shoulders are the sides of the yoke, balancing at the top of the chest cone and extending far enough beyond it to free the arm swing. The chest cone echoes the shape of the lungs inside it, not the shoulder girdle outside it. The muscles from which the shoulder girdle hangs extend from the head and neck to the shoulder blades (scapulae) in the back, and to the clavicles in front. The trapezius muscles aid in holding the spine, head, shoulder, arm and upper ribs in alignment. Connection of the shoulder girdle with the head rather than with the chest converts a side-load into the easier top-load.

The tip of the shoulder hangs easily, below the ear lobe. The shoulder girdle supports the arm, which is attached to the shoulder blade (scapula). The head of the upper arm bone (humerus) fits into a socket which is shallower than the hip socket, and the capsular ligament is very loose, to give the arm free motion. The arm falls along the median line of the body, along the axis of gravity.

The triangular shoulder blades hang more to the sides of the chest than at the back and connect with the clavicles. Each clavicle acts like a yard-arm, keeping the shoulder joint away from the chest.

A spoke-like system of muscles converges at the shoulder. Nearly every bone in the trunk, from head to pelvis, furnishes surfaces for their attachments to the head, rib cage, spine, sternum, every vertebra from the axis to the sacrum, the muscle bands of the front abdominal wall, and the pelvis. This gives enormous power to the arms and hands for heavy work, and also for fine-motor movements. It also means that arm movement interacts with the legs, and even the feet.

The shoulder girdle should never sink upon the rib cage. The first four ribs should move easily, within their limits, to the side, back and front. The swinging arms should not impinge on the ribs. This protects the upper thorax for functioning of (1) blood vessels, especially around the aortic arch, where the blood leaves the heart, and (2) upper lungs.

Spine. The spine is a flexible, segmented bony column. Since it has to move both itself and the body masses that are attached to it, the column is composed of four opposing curves. They are named for the anatomical areas in which they occur: cervical, thoracic, lumbar and pelvic. The third cervical, fourth lumbar, and sixth, seventh, eighth and ninth thoracic are the vertebrae where the curves reverse, and are thus the most vulnerable places places along the spine. Viewed from the side, it is a long S-curve, actually two S's. See pages 23 and 24 for illustrations.

In the human spine the bodies of the vertebrae are the principal weight-receiving parts of the body. Each vertebra must carry the accumulated weight carried by all those above it. To meet this load, the vertebrae are bigger in all dimensions toward the base of the column. Viewed from front or back, the spine is a column, incrementally wider toward its base, like a tall, thin pyramid, or the Washington Monument. At the top, the first cervical vertebra, the atlas, supports the base of the skull, and at the lower end, the fifth lumbar vertebra lies in the pelvic base.

The vertebrae are linked and separated by intervertebral discs. The discs together fill about one-quarter of the length of the column. This system, with its supporting ligaments and muscles, stabilizes the spine and enables it to bear weight in the upright position.

The five areas of the spinal column are the following:

1. Seven cervical vertebrae in the neck. (Cervix — cervical, means "neck.") The cervical curve is the shallowest. The cervical spine holds the head, and provides support for the chest, shoulders and arms, which hang from the neck muscles. The head is balanced centrally on the top vertebra, the atlas.

2. Twelve thoracic vertebrae in the upper back. The thoracic curve is much deeper than that of the cervical spine, though it does not appear externally to be. Its length, its lateral symmetry and the front-to-back symmetry that the ribs and the sternum share give it its strength. The ribs extend from the thoracic vertebrae to the sternum, or breastbone. (Sternum means chest in Greek. Thorax means chest in Latin.) The thoracic cage holds the heart, lungs and upper digestive system.

3. Five lumbar vertebrae. These are the largest and deepest vertebrae, forming the most flexible portion of the spine, very deepset into the trunk, below the ribs. The lumbar spine is relatively short and deep in proportion to its length. It is very powerful and drives the action of the whole torso. It dominates shoulder, arm and leg action as well.

4. Five sacral vertebrae. These vertebrae form a plate, the sacrum, to which the pelvic girdle is attached. The top of the sacrum is broader than the lumbar vertebrae, but it tapers in all dimensions toward the coccyx, forming the keystone of the pelvic arch. The sacral, or pelvic, curve is the sharpest of all. (Sacrum in Latin is literally a "sacred thing.")

The weight of the body mass on the sacrum is so great that its five vertebrae are fused into a single bony mass, and their curve is immovable. (In the newborn infant, the spine is straight and very flexible, and all joints are movable. The sacrum is fused by about the twentieth year.) From the sacrum the body weight passes through the rest of the pelvic arch to the heads of the femurs (thighs), and down the legs to the feet.

5. The coccyx, containing four or five small vertebrae, is lightly fused. The coccyx is the dwindling remnant of a pre-human

tail. Its curve continues downward and forward. The coccyx is a forlorn thing, and always needs to be sheltered. It is named for the Latin and Greek word for the beak of the cuckoo bird, whose shape it resembles.

We may think the spine is a shallow structure just below the surface of the back. Perhaps this is because the only parts of it that we can feel are its "spines" down the middle of the back. The fact is that at all levels the spine is nearly centered in the body from front to back. At the top, the front of the atlas is just back of halfway between the front and back of the head. The lumbar spine, with all its heavy muscles and ligaments, occupies one-half of the volume of the lumbar segment and constitutes more than half of its weight. This is because the soft viscera in front are so much lighter than bone.

Proper alignment of the spine requires bilateral symmetry (not scoliosis). It also requires balance of the small muscles along the spine that align the vertebrae. Finally, it requires maintenance of the front-to-back curves. Therefore, all muscles that tend to arch the back have complementary muscles that tend to bend it toward the front. In well-aligned posture, all these muscles are at ease. Defective posture, typically lordosis, which is excess lumbar curve, leads to habitually strained muscles and a lack of balance of the bones at the joints. Degenerative diseases such as osteoporosis also submit the spine to chronic muscle strain.

T'ai Ch'i. The ancient Chinese art of T'ai-ch'i is a system of flowing movements which integrate mind and body. In T'ai Ch'i one is relaxed. The head is held as if suspended from the ceiling. The mind concentrates on the top of the head.

Taoism. According to Taoist philosophy, good health derives from living harmoniously with the universe. The development and preservation of flexibility and relaxation bring us into this harmony. Flexibility and relaxation encompass the mind and spirit as well as the body to release the physical and mental rigidity that is the enemy of good health. Taoist techniques have proven beneficial to health for thousands of years.

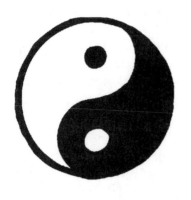

Illustration 73. YinYang

Taoism has no deity. It does not deal with evil, or salvation, but is simply the Tao: the Way. The closest text it has to a holy book is the TAO TE CHING.

Taoism was suppressed during the rule of the Mongols long ago, and has never recovered a broad following. Perhaps its most popularly visible symbol today is YinYang.

Thorax. The thorax is the chest and its contents. Its bones, the sternum, spine and ribs, form the rib cage. The rib cage protects the heart, lungs and upper digestive tract. The sides of the chest cavity are symmetrical, front to back and side to side. The top is surprisingly tapered, and described as cone-shaped, conforming to the shape of the tops of the lungs. The weight of the thorax is a frontal side-load on the spinal column, which means that it receives its main support from the thoracic spine.

Vertebra. See Spine.

Weight of a Body in Water. See Physics.

Yoga. Yoga is not a religion, as many people assume from its historic association with Buddhism, but neither is it merely sitting cross-legged on the floor. In its ancient form, yoga was called "the path of renunciation." The body was seen as an impediment on the path toward unity with the Divine.

More recently (corresponding to the Western sixth century A.D.), the "path of action" was conceived. Out of this grew Hatha Yoga, which, in an oversimplification which I shamefully acknowledge, honors the body as the true path to the Divine.

Some Hatha Yoga schools today emphasize only the meditational component of yoga. They find the cross-legged seated position enhances meditation, but pay little or no attention to posture in relation to health. Other yoga schools concentrate solely on the physical aspects of postures and stretches. They acknowledge a powerful spiritual force, but leave it to the practitioner to waken to that force through the unity of the mind/body/spirit. The Eastern names given to many yoga postures point the way to their spiritual aspect.

When the non-physical currents in the body are disrupted, the result is physical or emotional stress, or both. The purpose of yoga is to release this stress and rewire the subtle currents. Many yoga practitioners find that yoga is also a positive experience for personal growth and spiritual awakening. It leads to inner peace and to integrity, clarity and compassion. It is a kind of journey, or path, to higher states of awareness. In this way it is both mysterious and profound.

Zen. In the wake of the second World War, Daisetz Suzuki introduced America to Zen Buddhism. Zen Buddhism is not a religion in the Western sense. It is not concerned with philosophy or theology. It does not conflict with or intrude on any religion one may practice.

Suzuki says, "it is almost impossible to talk about [Zen] Buddhism. So not to say anything, just to practice it, is the best way. Showing one finger or drawing a round circle may be the way, or simply to bow. *** [D]o everything without thinking about whether it is good or bad, and when you do something with your whole mind and body . . . that is our way."

SOURCES FOR ADDITIONAL READING

Chopra, Deepak, M.D. PERFECT HEALTH. Harmony Books, Crown Publishing Co.

Drake. THE ALEXANDER METHOD. Harper Collins

Feldenkrais, Moshe. AWARENESS THROUGH MOVEMENT. HEALTH EXERCISES FOR PERSONAL GROWTH. Harper & Row, 1972

Levine, Barbara Hoberman. YOUR BODY BELIEVES EVERY WORD YOU SAY. Aslan Publishing, 310 Blue Ridge Drive, Boulder Creek, CA 95006, 1991

Iyengar, B.K.S. LIGHT ON PRANAYAMA. Crossroads Press, 370 Lexington, New York, NY 10017

Liu, Da. TAOIST HEALTH EXERCISE BOOK. Paragon House, N. Y. 1991

Mehta, Shyan, Silva & Meera. YOGA THE IYENGAR WAY, Knopf

Schatz, Mary Pullig, M.D. BACK CARE BASICS. A DOCTOR'S GENTLE YOGA PROGRAM FOR BACK AND NECK PAIN RELIEF. Rodmell Press, Berkeley CA, 1992

STEDMAN'S MEDICAL DICTIONARY. Williams & Wilkins, Baltimore, MD

Stransky, Judith, with Robert B. Stone, Ph.D. ALEXANDER TECHNIQUE, THE JOY IN THE LIFE OF YOUR BODY. Beaufort Books., Inc. NY 1981

Suzuki, Shunryu, ZEN MIND, BEGINNER'S MIND. Weatherhill, Inc., New York

Todd, Mabel E., THE THINKING BODY. Princeton Book Company P.O. Box 57, Pennington, NJ 08534

And browse through your local library and bookstore.

RESOURCES

American Center for the Alexander Technique, Inc., 142 West End Avenue, New York, NY 10023. Telephone (212) 799-0468

Arthritis Foundation, P.O. Box 7669, Atlanta, GA 30357-0669

Feldenkrais Guild, P.O. Box 11145, Main Office, San Francisco, CA 94101.

Yoga Journal. P.O. Box 469018, Escondido, CA 92046-9018

LIST OF POSTURES AND STRETCHES

POSTURES

Mountain
Dinosaur
Alexander Technique
Lampshade

Arrow A
Arrow B
Suspended Zen
Alexander-Style Relaxation

STRETCHES

Half Moon
Arch/Slump
Twist, Mountain
Atlas Rocking
Crane
Axis Turning
Neck Bending
Pelvis Rock
Tree
Stork
Five Pointed Star
Prayer
Prayer Circles
Shrug
Shoulder Hinge
Street Light
Snake Charmer
Quadrilateral
Achilles Stretch A
Passive Straight Leg Raise
Active Straight Leg Raise
Passive Bent Leg Raise
Active Bent Leg Raise
Side Leg Raise
Cautious Back-Bend
Daring Back-Bend
Cat on a Wall

Hip Swings
Standing Triangle
High Step
Spider-Man
Achilles Stretch B
Spring-Board
Goose-Step
Side Leg Raise at a Wall
Front Leg Raise at aWall
Cat on a Noodle
Pendulum Front to Back
Pendulum Side to Side
Twist, Suspended
Arabesque
Triangle, Suspended
Diamond, Suspended
Twist, Kneeling
Triangle Split
Warrior
Tai Ch'i
Hip Press
Half-Yoga Sit
Ankle Sit
Tailor's Seat A
Cat
Tailor's Seat B.
Hip Hinges

LIST OF POSTURES AND STRETCHES. continued

Cobra
Leg Raise to Side, Reclining
Straight Leg Raise, Reclining
Knee Hug
Straight Leg Twist, Reclining
Bent Leg Twist, Reclining
Crossed Knee (Mild)
Crossed Knee (Strong)
Foot and Ankle Stretch
Wrist and Finger Stretch

Jaw Stretch
Half Dog
Cat in the Shower
Lengthening the Spine
Marsh Grass
Swaying to the Side
Inducing the Natural Curve
Swaying Front to Back
Good Neighbors

GENTLE MOVEMENTS

Swing to Sides
Swing Front to Back

Bicycle
Sit-ups, Suspended

COMPLEMENTARY PRACTICES

Body Awareness in Everyday
    Life
Stress Management
Progressive Muscle
    Relaxation Technique
Deep Breathing
Breathing Without Breathing
Paradoxical Breathing
Hissing

Head and Face Massage
Trapezius Massage
Abdominal Massage
Kidney Massage
Knee Massage
Meditation
Body Messages
Imaging, Visualization
Affirmations

LIST OF PHOTOGRAPHS

LIST OF DRAWINGS:

hunched, and the top rib canted toward the front. All of this has the effect of shortening the appearance of the neck.

11. Page 61. Top views of lampshade and thoracic skeleton including spine, ribs, clavicles, and scapulae. Front view of lampshade. The shade is balanced on the axis of gravity of the lamp, just as the shoulder/arm system is balanced on the axis of gravity of the body.

12. Page 64. Half-Moon

13. Page 65. Arch/Slump

14. Page 66. Twist, Mountain. Notice that head turns to left, feet turn to right.

15. Page 70. Neck Bending

16. Page 71. Psoas and iliopsoas muscles, front view of right side. Together they form a major muscle system in the interior of the abdomen, connecting the lower ribs and pelvis to the thigh.

17. Page 73. Tree

18. Page 74. Stork

19. Page 75. Five Pointed Star

20. Page 76. Movement of the shoulders in raising the arms. View a shows correct movement, and view b shows incorrect movement for yoga. Even though the figure can reach a little higher, the neck and shoulder muscles are constricted. Notice how much longer the neck is and how much more space there is between the head and shoulders in View a.

21. Page 77. Prayer

22. Page 78. Shoulder Hinge

23. Page 79. Street Light

24. Page 80. Snake Charmer. A series of four drawings guides you into this stretch.

25. Page 82. Quadrilateral

26. Page 83. Achilles Stretch A

27. Page 84. Passive Straight Leg Raise

28. Page 85. Passive Bent Leg Raise

29. Page 86. Side Leg Raise

30. Page 92. Arrow

31. Page 93. Cautious Back-Bend

32. Page 94. Daring Back-Bend

33. Page 95. Cat on a Wall

34. Page 96. Hip Swings

35. Page 97. Standing Triangle

36. Page 98. High Step

37. Page 99. Spider-Man

38. Page 100. Achilles B

39. Page 101. Spring-Board

INDEX

WATERYOGA

SUGGESTION BOX

See other side for Order Form.

Because WATERYOGA presents a new exploration into bodywork and wellness, I am eager for your response. Whether you have found something as serious as a misstatement of anatomy or physics, or as innocent as a typographical error or misspelled word, please let me know.

I also hope you'll send me your thoughts, comments, suggestions and criticisms. They will be gratefully considered for future printings.

Jill Coleman

c/o Eglantine Press
10707 Sprinkle Lane
Owings Mills, MD 21117
U.S.A.

Your Name _____

and address _____

(optional) _____

WATERYOGA
ORDER FORM

Please send me _____ copies of WATERYOGA, by Jill Coleman.

Name:_____

Address: _____

City, State, Zip Code: _____

Phone No. (optional) (_____) _____

One copy @ $17.95 $_____.____
                    Plus
____Additional copies @ $12.95   _____.____ = $_____.____

Maryland residents add 5% sales tax   _____.____

Shipping: first copy @ $4.00   _____.____

Shipping: _____ additional copies @ $2.00 each   _____.____

TOTAL: $ _____.____

Enclosed is my check or money order. Please allow three weeks for delivery.

Dealers: please inquire about dealer discounts.